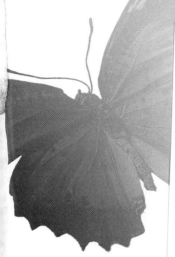
ip and
nent

ach

Editors:

Elaine McNichol and Susan Hamer

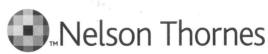

Nelson Thornes
a Wolters Kluwer business

Published in 2007 by:
Nelson Thornes Ltd
Delta Place
27 Bath Road
CHELTENHAM
GL53 7TH
United Kingdom

07 08 09 10 11 / 10 9 8 7 6 5 4 3 2 1

A catalogue record for this book is available from the British Library

ISBN 978 0 7487 9767 7

Cover photograph/illustration by Stockbyte RF (NT)
Illustrations by Florence Production Ltd, Stoodleigh, Devon
Page make-up by Florence Production Ltd, Stoodleigh, Devon

Printed and bound in Slovenia by DELO tiskarna by arrangement with Korotan-Ljubljana

Acknowledgements

With thanks to the following for permission to reproduce copyright material in this book:

The Leadership Qualities Framework © Crown copyright 2002, p. 35.
Creative Health Care Management for the Commitment to my Co-worker © statement, pp. 99–100.

Every effort has been made to contact copyright holders. The publishers apologise to anyone whose rights have been inadvertently overlooked, and will be happy to rectify any errors or omissions.

Contents

Acknowledgements

We have been planning this book for a long time and as such it goes deeply into our academic and practice interests. We both share a passion for learning and there have been times when we have been frustrated by our inability to support individuals, teams and organisations in applying knowledge faster in order to effect improvement in health services.

Like all practitioners, we have reflected on, refined and improved our practice. The people we work with have given us feedback, shared their ideas and challenged us to have rigour in our thinking. To all these individuals we owe a debt of gratitude. This text is a synthesis of a complex field of enquiry which we have ourselves had to organise and apply. We are sharing with you what we and our co-authors have found most useful. Many of the tools are good friends, and we are confident that they will help you move forward as you develop your own skills in the critical area of leadership and management.

We would also like to acknowledge the support and encouragement of those family and friends who even as they say 'go for it' know that it will mean fewer home-cooked meals and slightly dustier houses; fortunately, we have never been known for being domestic goddesses and are better known for our passion for great patient care. We promise to continue to try to do better on both.

Elaine and Susan

Preface

The purpose of this book is to provide an overview of leadership and management to those of you who are new to the health care field or to those lifelong learners who wish to refresh their understanding and skills.

Leadership and management is a large and complex field of enquiry with many conflicting views. We have made no attempt to provide you with a comprehensive account (that would be a very large book indeed); instead we have chosen to focus on those applied areas of knowledge that we know will be helpful to you, as they have been for us and the teams with whom we have worked.

The 3-dimensional approach to leadership and management offers you a framework with which to structure your thinking and reflections. Unfortunately, we are unable to present any elegant solutions that you can go away and apply with predictable outcomes. Rather, we hope that you will use the contents of this book to stimulate your own thinking; combine what you read with your own personal experiences, and in time develop your own theory of leadership and management.

Each chapter has a range of features designed to help you. As some of the terms that we use will be new or used in unfamiliar ways, there is a **Keywords** section in the margins, where you will be able to read a more detailed definition of words used. To help clarify the key points, each chapter begins with some clear goals – **Learning outcomes** – and ends with **Rapid recap** questions to review your understanding.

You will be encouraged to think about new ideas and to test your understanding in **Over to you** and **Reflective activities.** This gives you the chance to weave new ideas into your previous understanding and consider applying them in your practice. Many of these activities could also provide the basis for a study day or supervisory session with other team members. Indeed, we would actively encourage you to discuss some of the ideas raised with others as this will help your own thinking to develop more rapidly. For this reason, we have also written the chapters in such a way that you will be able to dip in and out and revisit some of the ideas as you change in your role and professional development.

Another feature that we have all enjoyed is the **Case studies,** including those where a **Health professional speaks**. These are real examples and should hopefully reassure you that this is an area where we are all on a learning journey.

As mentioned earlier, leadership and management is a large field of study; key areas where there is important work are therefore referenced at the end of each chapter, and most of the chapters include an **Evidence base** feature, with recommendations for further reading; suggestions for additional web-based resources are also given in some sections.

There are many ways in which leadership and management can help us gain a better understanding of how we work and how the health systems in which we practise change and develop. With an increasingly robust evidence base available, we also know that the quality of leadership and management has a direct impact on patient outcomes. Leadership and management have become a fundamental skill set for all health professionals. However, knowing where to begin to develop your skills is a real challenge. In Chapter 1, we look at the changing context of health, as this is a key area for consideration before you decide which aspects of leadership and management you may prioritise for development. Understanding the important role of culture and the key policy drivers will enable you to step back and be more purposeful in your approach. In Chapter 1, we also introduce you to the 3-dimensional model of leadership and management in health systems, and this forms the framework for the following chapters.

In Chapter 2, we look in much closer detail at you as a leader. The chapter provides an overview of leadership theory, and encourages you to reflect on your own behaviours. In particular, it considers the use of power, and encourages you to unlock your potential by perhaps seeing yourself differently. Chapter 3 follows a similar layout: we first of all look at the key management theories and those management behaviours that are known to be essential in order to be effective. A range of development options is also presented. Having secured a solid foundation of self-knowledge and awareness, we can then move forward to consider how we contribute and operate in a team.

Teams are an essential ingredient in so much of our lives, as families, socially and in work organisations, and Chapters 4 and 5 look at effective team leadership and management, respectively. A wide range of aspects of team behaviour is considered: how teams communicate; their different shapes; how they learn; why they under-perform and where they fit into organisational design. Once again, there are many opportunities for you to reflect on your own team and gain insights into how you could develop it with more effective leadership and management strategies.

Perhaps a unique feature of this book is its focus on the patient. Patient-centred care should be at the heart of all our leadership and management endeavours, yet perhaps is still too often an afterthought. In Chapters 6 and 7, we look at patient-centred care from a variety of perspectives and describe the progression from professionally centred to patient-centred health services. These chapters also cover how to obtain and use meaningful feedback from patients and how to deal with challenging patient situations without reverting to disempowering activities; they will encourage you to consider what the future for patient-centred leadership may look like.

Finally, we walk forward in Chapter 8 to imagine the future; we look at some of the current trends in health care leadership and management where the research is less developed but the ideas look very exciting. We consider just what you will need to do to be well prepared to respond to the opportunities that these futures may present.

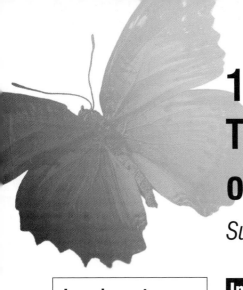

1
The changing world of health

Susan Hamer

Learning outcomes

By the end of this chapter you should be able to:

★ Understand how key trends influence health systems

★ Understand why you perceive change both positively and negatively

★ Identify the four elements of the McNichol and Hamer 3-dimensional model of leadership and management

★ Recognise the relationship between work–life balance and effective leadership and management.

Introduction

If you were to have a conversation about health anywhere in the world, I have no doubt that before long the terms 'leadership', 'management' and 'patients' would soon crop up. These terms would be closely associated with the expression of some goal, dream or target for improving a health outcome. Indeed, the only constancy in health services seems to be change: people discuss how to make change happen; how fast it should be and who should be carrying it out.

This chapter looks in detail at this changing world of health. It will seek to map out key trends that are a consequence of broader societal shifts and changing public expectations. Understanding this context is an important element of developing your own sense of direction and, consequently, the role that you would wish to play as a leader and manager.

What is changing?

Look around you and think of all the things that you have changed in your life in the last six months. Your response may include significant aspects of your life, such as your job, where you live and relationships, and it will certainly include clothes and music. In Table 1, you will see a list of some of the larger changes happening in society that have significant consequences for all of us and affect our jobs, lives and even the weather!

Table 1.1 Types of change affecting society

Source of change	Nature of change
Human	Changing demography Urbanisation Migration Refugees
Environment	Climate change Biodiversity Disasters
Political systems	Human rights Democracy Corruption
Employment	Adult learning Intergenerational working Recycling jobs (lost and created) Changing business models
Resources	Water Energy Food
Communication	Transportation Internet
Culture	Science Religion Drugs Consumerism
Health	HIV/AIDS Malaria Global pandemics

Reflective activity

Consider Table 1.1. Think of how these different changes affect different people. What you may perceive as a negative could be an exciting opportunity for someone else.

● Today, it is not uncommon to have a health service globally networked; for example, X-rays taken in one country may be reported on from another country, perhaps on the other side of the world. What do you think about that?

● In the past, a career in the health service meant doing the same job for 25 years, then retiring and getting a pension. Individuals entering the workforce today are now looking at 50 years in active work. What will that mean in terms of health, employment, **culture**, communication and policy?

● Do you talk about these things with colleagues?

⚷ *Keywords*

Culture
Comprises the informal psychological and social aspects of an organisation that influence how people think

Keywords

Health system
The people, institutions and resources that operate as a whole to provide health care and improve the health of the population served

Needs
Are anything that is necessary but lacking

Health workers
Are all people primarily engaged in actions with the primary intent of enhancing health

Lifelong learning
'Those forms of teaching and learning that equip individuals to encounter with competence and confidence, the full range of working, learning and life experiences' (Kogan, 2000)

The health services that we work in are not immune from these changes as we can see from Table 1.2, and the driving forces for change do present us with some real challenges. Many of the existing systems were designed for a world – and workforce – that no longer exists. As **health systems** seek to respond to these contemporary **needs**, then so too does the world of work. This will call for us to be more active in seeking to understand what is required of us as individuals, working in teams and in increasingly complex organisations.

In the past, the skills to respond to these challenges could be learnt in a more measured way; now, the pace of change requires a swifter learning response. In anticipation of this there has been an unprecedented investment in ensuring that **health workers** have more ready access to training and education opportunities associated with an expectation of **lifelong learning**. Indeed, many of you reading this book may already have worked in health in the past and are seeking to refresh your own skill set.

Table 1.2 Forces driving the workforce

Driving forces			Workforce challenges
Health needs profile ——→	——→		**Numbers**
Changes in the age of the population The prevalence of different illnesses Epidemics			Skills shortages Over supply Skill mix Generational balance
Health systems ——→	——→		**Distribution**
Funding for health Technology Consumer expectations			Primary/secondary International migration
Context ——→	——→		**Workforce conditions**
Health service reform Workforce changes and education Worldwide sharing of information			Pay and rewards Lifelong learning Workplace safety

Reflective activity

Think of a new skill that you have recently learnt. Did learning mean that you had to stop doing something you had been doing before? Did you have to go on a course or did somebody demonstrate the skill to you? Did you need to read and write something? Do you know how you best learn new things? Is it easier to do it the old way? What helps you do it the new way?

O━━ᴛ *Keywords*

Data
Are raw symbols and facts

Information
Comprises data that make
a difference

Knowledge
Is information with a
purpose

**Leadership and
management**
Are activities that result in
action through a series of
negotiations which aim to
resolve the needs and
wants of care providers and
care receivers

We now have a much better educated workforce than ever before, but
knowing what to learn also becomes more complex. The explosion of
data and **information**, as evidenced by the Internet, can mean that
developing a **knowledge** base for professional practice has also become
more confusing and complex. We do, however, know from the research
literature that competence (the ability to perform work activities to the
standard required) in certain skill sets is associated with improved health
outcomes for patients.

This is why, when you discuss health care, **leadership and
management** are in the foreground; they make a difference. Good
leadership and management save lives and poor leadership and
management are associated with higher levels of morbidity and
mortality.

Strengthening health systems

The scientific advances that we see on an almost daily basis have led to
significant improvements in health worldwide. Yet, at the same time,
there are some major reversals. In the United Kingdom, we have seen
increases in childhood infectious diseases, such as measles, and, despite
a much greater understanding of nutrition, obesity is now posing a major
threat to the health of a whole generation in mature Western
democracies. Life expectation in some of the poorest countries is half
the level of the richest, owing to diseases such as HIV/AIDS and malaria.
Knowing what may cause a disease and having the cure for it is simply
not enough. As the World Health Organization (WHO) noted
controversially in a report about the state of the world's health:

> the world community has sufficient financial resources and
> technologies to tackle most of these health challenges yet today
> many health systems are weak, unresponsive, inequitable – even
> unsafe.
>
> WHO (2006, p. xv)

Reflective activity

Look again at the above quote from the WHO and think of recent news items
about health. Do you agree that we have enough money to tackle many of the
world's big health problems? Do you think that more money means better health?

It would appear obvious that failing to use available scientific evidence to
improve health is a waste of money and can lead to harmful practice.
That may mean stopping harmful interventions (the rise in caesarean

sections) as well as adopting new ones (the use of low-dose aspirin to prevent heart disease). So why is the gap between knowledge and practice so large? Why don't we as health workers rapidly incorporate best practice into our daily activities? Have we over-focused on technical competence and know-how at the expense of those skills that enable the system to work? As is sometimes said, 'the operation was a great success but the patient died!'

The World Health Organization has been working for many years to understand and strengthen health systems in order to reduce global disparities in health. In a comprehensive review of the current state of global health research carried out in 2004, it identified the following main points:

- Science must help to improve health systems. It should not focus solely on advancing academic knowledge or confine itself to producing new drugs, diagnostics, vaccines and medical devices.

- Biomedical discoveries cannot improve people's health without research to find out how to apply them specifically within different health systems and contexts.

- Health systems must interact closely with health research systems to generate and use knowledge for their own improvement.

- An environment conducive to evidence-informed health policy and practice should be created. To achieve this, the producers and users of research should work closely together to shape the research agenda and to ensure that research is used to improve health.

- Health systems research suffers from a poor image and has been under-funded compared with biomedical research despite widespread recognition of its importance. More funds are needed to develop new methodologies and **innovation** to deal with the changing environment within which health systems currently operate

(WHO, 2004, p. xv).

Clearly, the WHO sees that there is much to be gained by strengthening health systems and that, as health systems are essentially a people-intensive service, a fundamental goal must be the development of a capable and motivated workforce. As the report notes, the workforce is 'the human link that connects knowledge to action' (WHO, 2004).

Understanding this means that wherever you are in the health system you have a range of responsibilities for improving it (a point we will return to in the following chapters), but this view is clearly at odds with one held too commonly by those individuals in some systems who believe that 'it's just a job and I have no **power** to change things'.

Keywords

Innovation

Is the process of converting knowledge and ideas into better ways of doing business, or into new or improved products and services

Keywords

Power

'Power is the ability to do something or to act in a particular way' (Oxford University Press, 2001)

Evidence base

In order to provide you with a comprehensive overview of the challenges facing world health and some suggestions on how the world can begin tackling these, starting at the level of the individual, we recommend that you read the World Health Organization's (2004) *World Report on Knowledge for Better Health: Strengthening Health Systems*. It can be accessed at: www.idrc.ca/en/ev-91519-201-1-DO_TOPIC.html.

Over to you

This team exercise is called a PEST. It will help you to identify larger issues that you will have to respond to as a team. On a large piece of paper, draw a square and divide it into four quarters, as shown in the figure. Label the quarters: political; economic; social and technological, respectively.

Political	Economic
Social	Technological

A PEST

Think of the challenges facing the team that you currently work with. Encourage colleagues to shout out ideas and write them in the appropriate quarter; stand back and lead a discussion about how, as a team, you could change the system; how you can influence and be better prepared for the challenges that you can see.

This is a useful exercise for you and the team to do at least once a year.

Disseminating innovation – is change too slow or too fast?

> ### Reflective activity
>
> Not long ago it was very common for most abdominal surgical procedures to require a large incision, which resulted in a stay of several days in a hospital and a range of possible side effects. Now, a large amount of surgery is done using laparoscopic procedures, and the patient is treated as a day case. What have the consequences of this change been for patients, surgeons, nurses, and employers? This is an area where the adoption of new practice has been swift. Can you think why that might be the case?
>
> Jot your ideas down because we will be returning to this issue.

In health care, invention is hard but dissemination is even harder.

Berwick (2003)

Keywords

Values
These underpin your beliefs and behaviours; values help to provide you with direction at difficult times as they are the standards by which you can make judgements regarding actions and decisions

In part, understanding how to support change in health systems involves knowing when to change and what actions to take. The study of the take-up of new ideas has quite a long history, particularly in the social sciences. However, across a number of studies there are three key areas that relate to how fast an idea is spread and subsequently adopted:

- perceptions of the innovation (Box 1.1)
- characteristics of the people who adopt the innovation (Box 1.2), and
- context features especially involving leadership, management, communication and incentives (Box 1.3).

Box 1.1 Perception of the innovation

Will the change benefit me? If yes, more likely to adopt

Does it match my **values** and beliefs? If yes, more likely to adopt

Generally, simple innovations spread more quickly than complicated ones

Can I test in a small way before adopting it? If yes, more likely to adopt

Can I see someone else do it? If yes, more likely to adopt

Box 1.2 Characteristics of the individual

Rogers (1995) classified adopters of innovation into five groups:

- Innovators 2.5% – adventurous, tolerant of risk, like new things, look for new things
- Early adopters 13.5% – opinion leaders, locally well connected, cross-pollinate, speak to innovators
- Early majority 34% – learn from people they know well, like to hear about ideas relevant to current and local problems
- Late majority 34% – look to early majority for what is safe, look for local proof, will adopt when innovation appears the new status quo
- Traditionalists 16% – point of reference is the past, swear by established and tested

Box 1.3 Contextual factors

How easy is it for innovators to grow? (Especially as they may take more risks and have more failures)

How easy is it for innovators to network with early adopters?

Are there flexible decision-making styles that encourage a broad range of ideas?

As we can see, understanding the spread of change starts to signpost key behaviours that may enable you to support the change process in a health system. Much of the research literature in this field is descriptive and observational; however, leaders in this field of enquiry are increasingly confident that the research does support some conclusions. Berwick (2003) has identified seven rules:

1 Find sound innovations.
2 Find and support innovators.
3 Invest in early adopters.
4 Make early adopter activity observable.
5 Trust and enable reinvention.
6 Create slack for change.
7 Lead by example.

> ## Reflective activity
>
> Look again at your answers to the previous reflective activity on page 7. Did you identify some of the points that you see listed in Boxes 1.1–1.3? If you have tried to change something in the past and been unsuccessful, do you now have an idea as to why it may not have worked?
>
> What sort of an 'adopter' are you? Do you let other people know how you react to new ideas so they can best support your learning?

The changing world of work

Looking at the changing context in which health services are delivered, it is clear that, ideally, changes aimed at improving care are best initiated by health workers themselves, namely you. You will be working as part of a team, maybe several teams. However, perhaps like me you will also have commitments elsewhere: I am a wife, a mother, a daughter, and these roles also require skills of leadership and management. So it is useful to recognise that many of the ways in which we deal positively with change at work could be equally applicable to home-life activities and can be shared with family and friends.

We do know that stress can be generated when roles come into conflict. Levels of ill health, both physical and psychological, and associated sickness absence are high among those working in health care. Poor health in the workforce can clearly mean that both quality and quantity of patient care can be reduced (Borrill *et al.*,1996; Borrill *et al.*, 2002).

In an extensive review of the relevant literature, Michie and Williams (2003) identified the following key work factors associated with poor health in the workforce:

- long hours worked
- work overload and pressure (and the effects of these on home life)
- lack of control over work
- lack of participation in decision-making
- poor social support
- unclear (poor) management and unclear work roles.

Historically, responsibility for 'getting the balance right' has been placed at the feet of individual health workers. Now, however, there is a much greater appreciation that health organisations need a coherent strategy for the prevention, management and treatment of work-related stress. Nevertheless, achieving this system-wide change requires genuine commitment from all members of the health system. This in turn needs approaches to change that are reflected upon, planned, implemented and reviewed (Cottrell, 2001).

Reflective activity

Currently, in Canada there are about four nurses per doctor, whilst Mexico has fewer than one nurse per doctor.

Do you think this is a good thing? Could it create stress in the workplace?

If you were part of a health team in Mexico, how would you need to work differently?

When you look around your own team/organisation, do you think there are places where there are too many of one sort of health professional and not enough of another? For instance, at my local general practice it is easier to see a doctor than a nurse. What should we/you do about this?

Just how easy is it to get the right worker, with the right skills in the right place doing the right things? Is a certain level of workplace stress an inevitable consequence of a rapidly changing system?

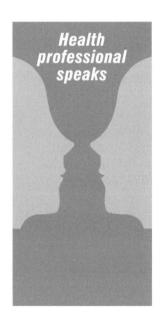

Health professional speaks

Health visitor

I am a health visitor on a busy inner city estate; we had traditionally always had four health visitors in our team. However, one left and, despite repeated advertising, one year on we still had not found a replacement. The work pressure was high and worrying. One day it came to a head with a complaint from a mother. Her complaint was not unreasonable, and as a team we had to look at how we were working and ask some fundamental questions. Why did we need four health visitors? That was a historical pattern, yet our work had changed hugely. Who else out there could help us achieve our goals? What was the key health prevention work we wanted to promote? In the end, our solution was to recruit two nursery nurses who, as part of their role, trained and supported a group of mothers to run their own groups to promote healthy eating and breastfeeding. Our workforce increased in size several fold but not in cost. The empowerment in the local community was brilliant to see. This change enabled the three health visitors to focus on the more complex cases which better used their skills. I am sorry that it took a crisis to make us look at our practice. We have since set regular time aside and invited a member of staff from a local university to act as a critical friend as we plan and develop our services.

Many of the challenges facing the workforce have the potential to create real problems (some would argue that they already have, if you consider skill shortages in midwifery care and mental health services). So how do you make sure that you are best able to meet this challenge, and, in your role as a leader/manager, how do you develop an enabling environment for others that helps manage both your and their stress levels? This is the foundation of the following chapters, where we look in detail at you as a leader and at working in a team and being responsible and accountable for patient-centred services.

> ## Reflective activity
>
> I would like you to think of a time when you had a really good day at work. What happened that day? What did people say and do? What was happening in the environment? Try to complete the following statements.
> - I am most confident when I . . .
> - I learn most easily when there is . . .
> - I am most receptive to new ideas when I . . .
> - I ask my best questions when I . . .
> - I listen most effectively when I can . . .

As referred to earlier, research suggests that when health workers do their best work it is seldom driven by financial incentives alone. There are other aspects of their work environment that are more important. These aspects are detailed in the box below. The skills associated with the creation of this important environment for both health workers and their patients, I have termed purposeful leadership and management.

Good job factors

You are more likely to do a good job when:
- There is a clear sense of vision and purpose
- You feel valued and recognised for your contribution whatever your job
- You feel engaged in the decision-making processes (an atmosphere of openness)
- Teamwork is encouraged
- Supervision is readily available
- Feedback is part of the culture, with rewards available for good performance
- Innovation and creativity are supported

Purposeful leadership and management

Perhaps as you considered the list in the box above, you were thinking, 'Well that's good in theory. But, when the pressure is on to improve results fast, then, the task tends to dominate all activities.' You will often hear people say that what gets done is what is measured. Indeed, there will be times when an emphasis on results may ensure the survival of you, the team, and the organisation. In most cases, many of the demands that you accept as givens are actually discretionary in nature. As I am sure you have experienced, it can be all too easy to spend a day being highly reactive (fighting fires), which also makes the day fragmented and priorities harder to achieve. This imbalance of activity has to be temporary, and you will need systems in place to keep the balance right between your management (short-term actions) and leadership (bigger picture) behaviours. To do so, you will need to feel confident about dealing with competing demands, by setting boundaries and keeping to them.

Reflective activity

Do you ever go to bed thinking that you have achieved little in a day? Do you think you had the balance right between short-term, immediate and longer-term goals?

Leadership vs. management

Hopefully, from your short reflection during the previous exercise, you will be starting to ask yourself a question that has been the subject of many books and articles. That is, if getting the balance right is the answer then are some individuals naturals? Were they born to be good leaders/managers? Taking this one step forward, we could also ask if management/leadership is an art or a science.

Reflective activity

Was Florence Nightingale born to be a great leader/manager? Think about the portrayed image. It served an important purpose: its intent was to inspire others to serve whatever their birthright. In reality, Florence had had a very privileged childhood, was extremely well educated, moved in very influential circles, was trained from an early age to understand politics, and had some very powerful sponsors/mentors throughout her life.

The important point is that these are not mutually exclusive alternatives. As we see above in the case of Florence Nightingale, even if there was a certain aptitude (in her case for mathematics, writing, and organising supplies both human and material), these skills needed to be actively developed through a variety of planned learning experiences.

So having suggested that leadership – and management – is neither an art nor a science, and we are not born to be great at it but can develop greatness, is it possible to be a great leader and not a manager and vice versa? The distinction between leadership and management has been much debated. Generally, observers agree that there are some distinct differences between leaders and managers, mainly because of the roles

⊶ᴛ *Keywords*

Hierarchy
Is a structure that regulates the lines of responsibility and patterns of relationships between staff

that they take in groups and organisations. Having some sort of management **hierarchy** is one way of recognising and ordering the various levels of expertise and experience of the workforce, so, in consequence, by virtue of a role, you acquire management responsibilities. However, you are not a leader until your knowledge and skills in carrying out the functions of leadership are recognised and accepted by others (Adair, 2003a).

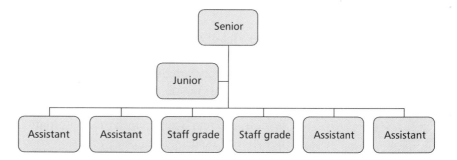

An example of a hierarchy of staff in a health care setting

Reflective activity

Effective management is seen as fundamental to the success and effectiveness of the organisation. However, what sustains organisations' performance in the long term is leadership.

Ashridge Management College (2006)

This is a bold statement, but do you agree? If so, can you give an example from your own experience as to why this may be the case?

Table 1.3 outlines commonly held views on the differences between leaders and managers.

Table 1.3 Differences between leaders and managers

Leaders	Managers
• Challenge	• Plan
• Develop a long-term focus	• Coordinate
• Are visionary	• Control
• Are people-focused	• Direct
• Ask what and why	• Ask how and why
• Mentor	• Are task-focused
• Innovate	• Organise
• Develop trust	• Present orientated
	• Are focused on the short term
	• Are reactive

While a lot of debate focuses on the differences between leaders and managers, if you look closely, as we noted at the beginning of the section, the distinctions are not so obvious. There are skills that unite the two roles, and it is possible to view many on a continuum. So, as you will see in the forthcoming chapters, although we make a distinction between leaders and managers in order to illuminate particular skill sets, they are not viewed as being in tension with one another but as complementary. There is no one right way to manage and lead. Your style will depend partly on the situation, partly upon the individuals you are dealing with, and partly upon your personality. A whole range of styles can be equally effective.

Leading and managing in complex health systems

Earlier on, we noted that we all have to contend with an unprecedented pace of change and an increasingly unpredictable organisation climate. As a result, leading and managing has had to change too: managing complexity, innovating and managing change are key current concerns, and several new theories have emerged to describe and explain these new behaviours. Complexity theory has been developed from a number of disciplines. It takes the view that the world is better described as a system (a network of elements that interact with each other) that is non-linear (so less predictable) and dynamic (changing continually). Kernick (2004) believes that the consequence of this is that organisations should be viewed as structures that not only bring people together to 'do a job' but also as places where people make sense of their lives. So that would mean that as managers and leaders we would be better thinking of an organisation as less like a machine and more like an ecosystem. The focus of management and leadership radically shifts, particularly in understanding the nature of relationships, how they organise and self-sustain.

Table 1.4 A comparison of two different ways of viewing organisations

Machine	Living system (complexity science)
• Focus is on the individual parts	• Focus is on the relationship between the parts
• The system can be understood by breaking it apart	• The system can only be understood as a whole
• The future is predictable and controllable	• The future is unpredictable but there are some knowns
• A change in a part of the system only affects those bits nearby	• A change in one part can change the whole system.
• Learning resides with the inventor	• Learning is distributed throughout the system

Reflective activity

Think of your current team as a machine. What terms would you use to describe it?

Did you think of it in parts, with pieces and inputs and outputs? What are the limitations of this way of thinking? Would a small part going wrong be noticed, and would it be possible for a small part to have a big impact on the machine?

Now think of your team as a living organism. What terms would you use to describe it?

If something small in the system changed, would there be ways in which the whole could respond to it?

Look at Table 1.4 and consider what this difference of approach may mean for you as a leader/manager.

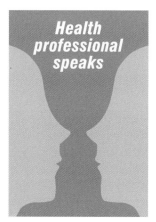

Health professional speaks

Housekeeper

Hello, I am Wendy, a housekeeper on a surgical ward. We recently had a change in management and all our shifts changed. It now means that I start later and can no longer help to feed the patients at breakfast time, a role I have been doing for years and like a lot. I also used to circulate the menus and check in with all the patients. Now I feel very rushed and that I have to rush the patients. I know that fewer patients are getting help. My frustration is that no one asked me about the possible consequences of the change; it was easy for me to see what was going to happen. I know we have to be efficient but sometimes changing little things can make a big difference to care, not always for the better.

As we can see, when changes are proposed, the impacts are frequently felt not just on what we do, such as introducing a new treatment, but on how we do it. Organisations change their management structures and team configurations on a very regular basis, and this produces a range of emotions and increasing levels of uncertainty and **ambiguity**.

Hodgson and White (2001) suggest that for the most part the previous experiences of leaders/managers have left them ill-prepared for people's lack of confidence when coping with change. They argue that in order to resolve this situation we need to:

- Achieve focus – focus on key strategic tasks and initiatives that everyone in the organisation must be aware of and subscribe to.
- Overcome fear of failure – upbringing and culture can make us risk adverse. As leaders we need to encourage experimentation and risk taking.
- Access your inner self – this urges us to use intuition and experience to spot ideas, trends and patterns that will help us make sense of things more quickly.
- Understand that simple questions lead to simple answers – as we can so easily become overloaded with information, simple, clear and concise communication about the direction and goals of the organisation is essential.
- Encourage energy and fun – an energised team is a creative and effective force.

Your role is helping others to find this motivating force within themselves.

It should now be evident why there is this increased emphasis on leading and managing both structure and cultures in organisations. As we saw earlier, there is a growing awareness that large structural reforms have not always delivered their intended impact, with services, staff and patients changing only a little. Cameron and Quinn (1999) suggest that it is the culture that is critical and that this determines the success of structural reforms.

Keywords

Ambiguity

Capable of more than one meaning

Evidence base

Read Knaus, W.A. *et al.* (1986) An Evaluated Outcome from Intensive Care in Major Medical Centres. *Annals of Internal Medicine*, **104**: 410–418.

A 3-dimensional approach to leadership and management

From our consideration of the changing context of leadership and management, it is clear that many of the skills required to be an effective leader/manager can be strengthened by your own willingness to learn and grow. However, that said, this is clearly a complex field of enquiry, and it is sometimes easier to represent complicated ideas using diagrams and **models**; this book is no exception. To help you think constructively about how you develop your approach to leading and managing in health systems, we have developed a model to help you to structure your action planning.

The McNichol and Hamer 3-dimensional model of health systems leadership and management is illustrated as a triangle with purposeful leadership and management as its central focus; the connecting sides are formed by **patient-centred care**, effective teams and understanding yourself. The whole triangle is encompassed in a circle to underline the importance of context to the achievement of purposeful leadership and management. The model suggests that these elements are interdependent and that any significant shift in any element will have significant consequences for the others; for example an increase in understanding yourself increases your capacity to support patient-centred care and contribute to effective teamworking.

⚷ Keywords

Model
Is a representation of a proposed structure that shows how it will work

Patient-centred care
At the most basic level, being patient centred means considering the values, preferences and needs of individual patients; at a more collective level, being patient centred means thinking about how patients or other members of the public can be involved in strategic planning and service development

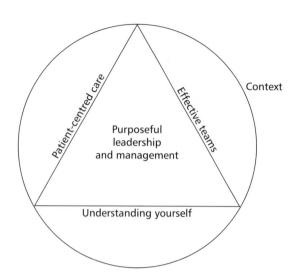

A 3-dimensional approach to leadership and management

Let's consider the four individual elements of the model in more detail.

Purposeful leadership and management

In order for health services to grow and develop to meet the changing expectations of the society we seek to serve, we have to adopt strategies that will enable a greater level of innovation and provide higher-quality services. To do this requires a significantly different leadership and management response. Indeed, those organisations where leaders do not respond to these new challenges will face serious problems and an uncertain future. The literature shows clearly that high-performance, innovative organisations require:

> inspirational leadership, stronger management skills, a highly motivated workforce, and the need for greater resource productivity.
>
> Department of Trade and Industry (2003)

It is this combination of attributes that we have termed 'purposeful leadership and management'. Namely, the ability to create a sense of vision in a rapidly changing health system; to motivate people and lead them through change; and to be able to be innovative in delivering services, developing new products and introducing new ways of working.

Patient-centred care

Patient-centred care works from the premise that patients know about their illness better than anyone else. If patients feel empowered, they will develop more choice and are more likely to take control of their own health. A self-management approach for patients with chronic diseases has been shown to improve health outcomes: for example in areas such as reduction of symptom severity, decrease in pain, reduced hospital admissions, fewer visits to general practitioners, and improved life control and activity.

Effective teamworking

Teams are the building blocks or connective tissue for all organisations. In a good team you are more likely to achieve the shared goals, and the social needs of individuals will also be met. According to Adair (2003b), high-performing teams have clear realistic objectives, a shared sense of purpose, make best use of resources, have an atmosphere of openness; are concerned to review progress; and have an ability to build on expertise to ride out organisational turbulence.

Understanding yourself

Much of our professional preparation is geared to self-sufficiency. We are in fact heavily dependent on others. Our own self-knowledge can be enhanced by our relationship with others. We need to understand how others see us. We may find it hard to share our uncertainty or anxiety about how things are going, but when we indicate what we really think about a situation we are likely to feel more secure.

The four elements described above are in constant dialogue with one another and will certainly change over time. It is not unusual for those new to a role to have a limited understanding of themselves. The value of this model is that it will help you to examine some key skills and behaviours and integrate your views on what leadership and management mean to you.

Reflective activity

Take some time now to draw the McNichol and Hamer model on a sheet of paper. As you start to think about the elements, draw the length of the line of the triangle to represent your level of confidence and understanding of that dimension.

If you feel that you do not have enough knowledge and skills in a dimension, make the line short. Finally, think about how big your context is. How well do you know what influences your wider world? Do you read an in-depth newspaper or journal on a regular basis?

Write the date on the paper as we will repeat this exercise later. It will be interesting to see if your triangle changes.

Conclusions

In today's increasingly uncertain, ever-changing and fast-moving world, organisations are relying more and more on individuals to come up with new ideas, to suggest new ways of doing things, to notice problems and to prevent them becoming serious. Innovation and change, whether in services, processes, technology or work practices, are designed by individuals. However, achieving the right environment, one in which individuals (health care workers or patients) feel confident enough to use their knowledge and offer their ideas, is a fundamental goal for leaders and managers.

Hopefully, by now you will be beginning to have a feel for the key elements that contribute to this leadership and management context. It is necessary for us all to stay aware of how larger changes in society have an impact on our day-to-day work; otherwise we are unable to respond, and we get locked into knee-jerk responses rather than devise plans that are well thought through. We also know that to effect positive change we must have a good understanding of some key skill sets, and leadership and management are at the core of these. However, the field of leadership and management is vast so it helps to have some sort of focus for our personal development, a framework. We have set out a framework – the McNichol and Hamer 3-dimensional model of leadership and management – which the following chapters will explore in more depth.

I believe that the health care context has never been so full of opportunities that are both challenging and exciting. There is a day-to-day balancing act to be struck between managing stability and knowing when to change. Nevertheless, in the quest to generate and support a culture of health systems improvement the following seven individual, team and organisational behaviours have been found to be most important:

- Put patients at the centre of everything you do.
- Believe in human potential.
- Encourage innovation and change.
- Recognise the value of learning.
- Strive for effective teamworking.
- Clearly communicate to everyone.
- Foster honesty and trust

  (NHS Modernisation Agency, 2004).

Finally, I would urge you to remember that you already have a wide range of leadership and management skills. Try to see yourself as a whole and to use skills that you have acquired throughout your life to date to help develop your own unique style of leadership and management. Although there is no right way to lead and manage, there are certainly better ways!

⚡⚡⚡⚡⚡**Rapid recap**

Check your progress so far by working through each of the following questions.

1. List six major trends that are currently actively influencing the development of health systems.
2. Describe two differences between a leader and a manager.
3. Describe four activities that would support the adoption of a new idea.
4. What would be four key features of a culture that fostered improvements in care?
5. List the four elements of the McNichol and Hamer 3-dimensional model of leadership and management.

If you have difficulty with more than one of the questions, read through the section again to refresh your understanding before moving on.

References

Adair, J. (2003a) *Not Bosses but Leaders: How to Lead the Way to Success*. Kogan Page, London.

Adair, J. (2003b) *The Inspirational Leader: How to Motivate, Encourage and Achieve Success*. Kogan Page, London.

Ashridge Management College (2006) *Leadership Learning Guide*, Ashridge.

Berwick, P.M., (2003) Disseminating Innovations in Health Care, *Journal of American Medical Association*, **289**(15): 1969–1975.

Borrill, C.S. *et al.* (1996) *Mental Health of Workforce of NHS Trusts: Final Report*. Institute of Work Psychology, University of Sheffield.

Borrill, C.S. *et al.* (2002) *The Effectiveness of Health Care Teams in the National Health Service*, Aston Business School, University of Aston.

Cameron, K.S. and Quinn R.C. (1999) *Diagnosing and Changing Organisation Culture: Based on the Competing Values Framework*. Addison & Wesley, Reading.

Cottrell, S. (2001) Occupational Stress and Job Satisfaction in Mental Health Nursing. *Journal of Psychiatric and Mental Health Nursing*. Apr **8**(2): 157–164.

Department of Trade and Industry (2003) *Innovation Review: Competing in the Global Economy, the Innovation Challenge*. DTI, London.

Hodgson, P., and White, R. (2001) *Relax, It's only Uncertainty*. Financial Times, Prentice Hall, Harlow.

Kernick, D. (2004) *Complexity and Healthcare Organisation*. Radcliffe Medical Press, Oxford.

Knaus, W.A. *et al.* (1986) An Evaluated Outcome from Intensive Care in Major Medical Centres. *Annals of Internal Medicine*, **104**: 410–418.

Kogan, M. (2000) Lifelong Learning in the UK. *European Journal of Education*, **35**(3): 343–359.

Michie, S. and Williams, S. (2003) Reducing Work-related Psychological Ill Health and Sickness Absence: A Systematic Literature Review. *Journal of Occupational and Environmental Medicine*, **60**: 3–9.

Moss Kanter, R. (1983) *The Change Masters*. Routledge, London.

NHS Modernisation Agency (2004) *Building and Nurturing an Improvement Culture*. NHS, London.

Rogers, E.M. (1995) *Diffusion of Innovations*, 5th edn. The Free Press, New York.

World Health Organization (2004) *World Report on Knowledge for Better Health: Strengthening Health Systems*. WHO, Geneva.

World Health Organization (2006) *Working Together for Health*. WHO, Geneva.

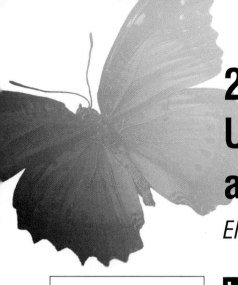

2
Understanding yourself as a leader

Elaine McNichol

Learning outcomes

By the end of this chapter you should be able to:

★ Briefly describe and discuss the different theories of leadership

★ Discuss the relevance of position and personal power to leadership

★ Identify and discuss key essential leadership behaviours

★ Apply an appropriate model of self-reflection to your own behaviours

★ Describe and discuss a range of developmental options in relation to leadership.

O—π *Keywords*

....

Work effectively

Working in a strong, credible and coherent way with other people to produce an intended or desired result

Four areas for self-knowledge

Introduction

In order to **work effectively** with others, you need, first, to be able to work effectively with yourself. This means understanding your beliefs and behaviours – and their impact on both your ability to be a great health professional – and the ability of those people working alongside you. In other words: 'leadership begins with greater self-knowledge' (McLean and Weitzel, 1992, p. 65). This chapter will take you on a journey of self-assessment, reflection and discovery in order to determine what sort of leader you are (your approach to leadership) and why leadership is relevant to you at all stages in your career. You will then be introduced to a range of practical steps that you can take to help you enhance your leadership ability.

McLean and Weitzel (1992, p. 67) suggest that in order to increase your level of self-knowledge and become better acquainted with yourself, you need to reflect on and analyse four areas: your interests, your abilities, your values and your needs.

Unlike wants, which are often emotionally laden, sometimes unreasonable and frequently too large to deliver on – 'I want to take the whole of August as annual leave' – needs are generally more specific, less demanding and often easier to meet. If you ask the question carefully – 'As a bottom line, what is it that you really need?' – the response – 'I have booked a holiday in Turkey for the first two weeks of August and I have no childcare cover for the third week' – makes the need explicit. Now you know that two weeks' annual leave

Interests	Abilities
Values	Needs

is required and can focus on the possibility of exploring some flexible working hours to help the person with their childcare cover.

> ### Reflective activity
>
> Spend 10 minutes listing at least 10 items in each quarter of the figure on page 23 and then ask yourself how the factors that you have identified:
> - influence your day-to-day practice
> - conflict with your day-to-day practice.
>
> For each area of potential conflict that you have identified, write down at least three options that you could choose to improve the situation.
> This exercise will provide a useful reference point for later activities.

Are you a leader?

> ### Reflective activity
>
> Are you a leader? Write down your initial thoughts and then reflect on their tone.

Perhaps you have written such things as:
- I am not old enough.
- I don't have enough experience.
- I haven't been doing the job long enough.
- It's not part of my role.

Or have you written any of the following?
- Yes, maybe – I often lead group exercises.
- I find it quite easy to persuade people around me to my way of thinking.
- I enjoy having ideas and (working with people), seeing how they could be taken forwards.

How you answered the above question will have been influenced by your perception of what makes a good leader, and whether you think being a good leader is connected to work or family role, maturity/age or experience.

Another question you might ask yourself is, 'Where are you when you demonstrate leadership behaviours?' Are you in the workplace, at home, within the community you live in, participating in a hobby or pastime or in some other arena or role?

These different responses reflect a key issue. Leadership is a process. It is about you as a person and the behaviours you engage in and how you manage your relationships with other people. It is *not* about position (Kouzes and Posner, 1997, p. xvii), job title, or how many years someone has been doing the job. Therefore *everyone* can be a leader and is in fact required to be in order to be an effective health care professional.

There are some fundamental assumptions about leadership (Management Research Group, 1992) that will underpin the content of this chapter:

- Effective leadership should be present at all levels in an organisation.
- There is no 'one right way' to lead.
- Effective leadership is based upon behaviour.
- Effective leadership behaviour depends upon the situation.
- Effective leadership is a reflection of how others perceive us.

So let us explore in more depth what it is that constitutes effective leadership.

Most effective/least effective leader

We have all experienced leadership: some that we felt was good and inspired us to greater things, and, on other occasions, leadership that we would not choose to repeat ourselves.

Reflective activity

Think about the people who you have worked with or observed and believe to be effective leaders. List in the table below what it is they do or did that, you think, makes them effective. If you believe that they are good communicators, then what exactly do they do? Do they, for example, explain things clearly, keep you informed, listen, etc.?

Table 2.1 Aspects of effective leadership

Effective leaders – What do they do?	How do you feel as a result? What is the impact on patient care?

Very often people stray into thinking about attributes rather than behaviours. The challenge is to describe the behaviours that result in the attribute that you are illustrating.

For example, when people are trustworthy they keep confidences, do what they say they are going to do and are consistent in what they say to different people.

Reflective activity

Now think about those people who, you believe, are or were ineffective leaders. We will assume that in many cases they did not do the things that you have identified in the above table. List in the table below what it is that they do or did that you think made them ineffective and the impact that this had on you.

Table 2.2 Aspects of ineffective leadership

Ineffective leaders – What do they do?	How do you feel as a result? What is the impact on patient care?

There are two key messages that should stand out from the above exercise.

1. Effective leadership is positively associated with health care staff feeling motivated, inspired and happy in their work. (Kreitner, 1995)
2. Effective leadership behaviours *plus* motivated, inspired and happy staff *equals* better quality care for patients (Smith, 1997; Salvage, 1999; Cunningham and Kitson, 2000). This is the single most powerful argument for improving the leadership abilities of all health care staff.

Position power and personal power

An important attribute of an effective leader is their understanding of and ability to use power in a positive and proactive manner. 'Power' is one of those words with which students and newly qualified or promoted staff often feel uncomfortable.

They are either nervous about using the power that naturally goes with their position, believe that they are relatively powerless or, conversely, are inexperienced in having power.

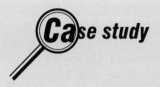

Understanding power

Sarah is 25-years-old, newly qualified and has been working in the day hospital for three weeks. Out of 10 staff, she is the second youngest. The remaining eight are aged between 28 and 59 years old and have worked there for between 1 and 15 years. On average, Sarah is in charge of three shifts out of five.

- What challenges do you think Sarah might be experiencing and why?
- What strategies would you recommend to overcome these challenges?

The understanding and appropriate use of power is an important feature of leadership. French and Raven (1968) describe two broad categories of power: position power and personal power.

Position power

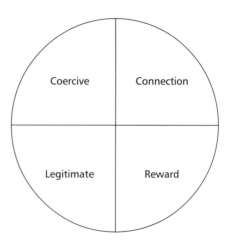

Position power

This type of power is associated with the position that you hold rather than the power that you possess as an individual: for example, a third-year student would hold more power than a first-year student; a charge nurse would hold more power than a staff nurse.

Connection power

Connection power refers to the contacts and connections that your position brings you that you would not otherwise have. Generally speaking, the more senior your position, then the more connection power you are likely to have. There are other sources of connection power, such as membership of trade unions or professional bodies.

Legitimate power

Legitimate power is the authority that is associated with the position you hold as opposed to your authority as an individual. Examples would include being able to agree study leave and annual leave or allocate work. This kind of power can be used in a 'neutral' way, or it can be used in either a coercive or rewarding manner in order to get people to do things for you.

Reward power

This is based on the ability to reward or favour – if you do this for me (cover this shift), then I will do this for you (agree your off-duty request) – there are overtones of bribery.

Coercive power

This type of power is more forceful and is based on the fear of penalties or punishments – if you don't do this for me (cover this shift), then I won't do that for you (agree your off-duty request) – here, there are overtones of blackmail.

Reflective activity

Can you identify a time when you either have or have not done something because of a person's ability to use their position power in a coercive or rewarding manner?

● How did you feel about it?

● Is it a position in which you often find yourself?

● When have you ever used your power in a coercive or rewarding manner (inside or outside of work)? What was your reason? Did you get what you wanted? How do you think the other person felt?

Personal power

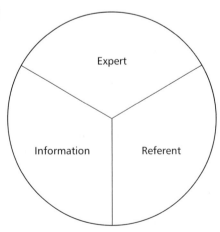

Personal power

In contrast, personal power is influence that you gain as an individual irrespective of your job title. You can be a ward housekeeper and have high personal power and, equally, you could be the chief executive and have low personal power.

Expert power

Expert power derives from having a high level of skill or technical knowledge in a particular field of practice or clinical procedure. People come to you for your expertise. Consequently, your views on issues related to your area of expertise (or sometimes even unrelated areas) carry more weight and influence. People with expert power are a great resource and can add value to any team. This is only true though, where the individual is willing to share their expertise. If the 'expert' is inhibited by a **scarcity mentality**, they are always mindful of whether they have given or done too much; to use a much-quoted metaphor, they are inclined to be 'half-empty glass' people as opposed to 'half-full glass' people. As sharing their expertise is thought to diminish their power rather than enhance it, they therefore 'hang on' to their expertise, and this power base can have a negative impact on others.

Referent power

This is very definitely a power that others confer on you: it is a reflection of their perception of how attractive a proposition it is to work with or be around you. If you have high referent power, then people will want to work with you and will volunteer to work alongside you or be part of a working group with you because it is a positive experience. Sometimes, referent power can just be a consequence of professional status (Marquis and Huston, 2003) and of the high regard in which the profession is held. Clearly, this makes the job of a leader easier as you are able to engage and develop followers.

Information power

Some people are always 'in the know'. They are up to date with the latest information; they even appear sometimes to be ahead of it! Their power comes from being very effective at proactively sourcing information rather than waiting for it to come to them. You will hear individuals with 'low information power' saying, for example, 'No one told me about it', 'I haven't time to read all these documents' or 'It's never been explained to me'.

Information power can also be subject to scarcity mentality. Because information and power have been inextricably linked through history, some individuals are reluctant to share or disseminate information, using it to control people and situations or to gain allies through selective disclosure.

⚷ *Keywords*

Scarcity mentality

Is a mindset in which a person believes that there is only so much that they can share, be that information, expertise, trust, or resources

Reflecti**Reflective activity**

Consider yourself and five other people with whom you work and complete the table below. Identify the power base of each one and make brief notes about how that influences the environment in your team or organisation.

Table 2.3 The impact of power base on communication and behaviour

The individual	Their power base(s)	Impact on communication and behaviour of others
Self		
Person 1		
Person 2		
Person 3		
Person 4		
Person 5		

Reflecti**Reflective activity**

Take some time to reflect on what types of power you use and to what extent. How strong is your personal power? Identify three ways in which you could strengthen your personal power and the impact that could have for you and those around you.

Whilst it is important to understand the position power that you may hold and how to use it appropriately, personal power is more influential and sustainable and therefore a critical component of effective leadership. However, the power bases described above are all related and can be present at varying levels within any one individual. Whether their use of power is perceived positively or negatively is determined in part by the individual's personal level of maturity and self-awareness and by the strength of their self-power base. In other words, the extent to which they are aware of their own power, their own strengths and weaknesses, and if they have a deep respect for themselves and for others (Farmer, 1993). Self-knowledge, therefore, becomes the primary source of power and is of greater importance than either positional or personal power. The more you know and understand yourself and take responsibility both for your behaviour and the consequences of that behaviour, the more likely you are to be a 'powerful' (strong) professional.

So, what is leadership?

Dictionary definitions favour a more traditional view of leadership that focuses on position power, using terms such as captaincy, control, rule and command. However, in both the wider literature and within health care, the prevalent understanding and perception of good leadership is couched more in terms of a balance between the use of position and personal power with increased emphasis on the characteristics of personal power such as guidance, direction, inspiration and **empowerment**. This is perhaps encapsulated by Handy (1993) who talks about a leader as being someone who shapes and shares the vision which then gives point to the work of others.

However, the literature contains a myriad of different leadership theories and perspectives. We have summarised the principal ones in Table 2.4 (see page 32).

Key leadership behaviours

As the table shows, there has not only been a gradual reduction in emphasis on the unilateral role of the leader but also the demystification of leadership as something that you either have or have not got. With the growing acceptance that there are identifiable effective leadership behaviours that we can all learn and practise, leadership has inevitably begun to be recognised as something that everyone can engage in, not just an identified few. This has resulted in increasing emphasis on the role of the followers to the extent that they are now viewed by many as co-leaders.

○━ᴨ *Keywords*

Empowerment
Is building the knowledge and confidence of individuals to enable them to participate effectively and assume authority

Evidence base

If any of the above theories is new to you or you would like to understand the theories in more depth, the following would be useful.

Buzan, T. (1981) *Make The Most of Your Mind*. Pan, London.
Cournoyer, P. (1990) The Nursing Shortage: Dynamics and Solutions. The Art of Creative Solutions. *Nursing Clinics of North America*. Sept. **25**(3): 581–586.
Crainer, S. (ed.) (1996) *Leaders on Leaders*. Institute of Management Foundation, Corby, Northants.
De Bono, E. (1967) *Uses of Lateral Thinking*. Penguin Books, London.
De Bono, E. (1985) *Six Thinking Hats*. Penguin Books, London.
Edmonstone, E. (2005) *Clinical Leadership – A Book of Readings*. Kingsham Press, Chichester.
Johnson, S. (1998) *Who Moved My Cheese?* Vermilion, London.

Table 2.4 Theories of leadership

Theory	Focus/assumptions
Great Man theory	Based on the belief that leaders are born (not made) with the innate qualities of leadership within them. Leadership was associated primarily with being male, military and Western
Trait theory	Built upon the principles of identifying the core behaviour traits displayed by born leaders. The goal being to be able to 'spot' those born to lead at an earlier age and place them into leadership positions. Stodgill (1974) summarises the predominate traits and skills identified
Behaviour theory	Began to focus on the behaviours of 'great' leaders rather than just their attributes, as the latter, e.g. integrity, were hard to measure
Transactional theory	Focuses on the relationship between the leader and the follower from the perspective of hierarchy and therefore position power. The relationship is viewed as a contractual one, whereby the follower receives rewards or recognition in return for loyalty to the leader. Tends to focus on day-to-day issues
Transformational theory	This also focuses on the relationship between the leader and the follower but from the perspective of personal power. It is underpinned by a greater emphasis on values and overall purpose and therefore focuses more on the long-term aim and how to work with people to achieve that aim. Principles of empowerment and maximising human potential are important
Situational theory	Proposes that there is no one right way to manage and that different situations require different interventions. An effective leader needs a flexible range of skills in order to best meet the inter-connecting needs of the leader, the follower and the task in hand within the surrounding environment (Handy, 1993). If any one of these factors changes, then so might the leadership intervention
Emotional intelligence (EI)	In this very specific theory, Daniel Goleman (1998) argues that whilst technical skills and cognitive ability are important, the defining characteristics of successful leaders are having a high level of emotional intelligence, the ability to work with others and to lead change. EI is characterised by high levels of self-awareness, self-regulation, motivation, empathy and social skill
Servant leadership theory	This signals a significant change in the perception of the role of the leader from being the person out front to someone who is much more aware of the inter-dependency of the roles of leader and follower. Leadership relates to service, being aware of and serving the needs of others in order for them, the team and the service to grow and flourish
Leaderful theory	This is part of an emerging theory known as 'dispersed leadership' where the role of leadership is separated from a person's position in the hierarchy. More than one leader can operate at the same time. The most appropriate person(s) for the situation take(s) the lead alongside the position leader. Leaders willingly and naturally share power with others. This paradigm re-defines leadership as a collective practice, that involves everyone and for which everyone has a potential ability to be involved (Raelin, 2003)

Reflective activity

Which one theory or combination of theories given in Table 2.4 best fits your perspective of effective leadership? Now consider the following:

- How is your perspective of effective leadership reflected in what you say and do?
- Identify at least three robust examples to illustrate this point.

So, if leadership is not about position or title but about what someone demonstrates through their actions and behaviours, then, whilst some people may have a natural flair for leadership, others can learn and develop relevant behaviours and skills in order to demonstrate more effective leadership.

Leadership models and frameworks

Keywords

Validated

As a result of research, there is substantial evidence that will corroborate that the tools do what they say they do

The literature contains a number of leadership models and frameworks that have grown out of the major theoretical perspectives. Some have been well researched and **validated**, whereas others are derived more from observation and experience and provide an easy-to-use checklist or, in some cases, almost a 'mantra'.

The following is a good example.

The Leadership Effectiveness Analysis™ (Management Research Group 1992) is a robust 360° analysis tool that identifies 22 leadership behaviours within 6 specific areas of leadership activity.

These include:

- creating a vision – showing enthusiastic commitment with an imagination and potential for independent thinking fully focused on current and future tasks, problems and opportunities

Keywords

Persuasion

Is an ability to influence the actions of others through one – or a combination of two or more – of the following – reasoning, argument, enthusiasm and commitment

- developing followers – having the ability to influence and use **persuasion** so that others respond positively to their ideas and efforts, through the strength of their logic, insight, imagination and communication skills
- implementing the vision – being able to communicate the part that others will play, delegate those parts, set standards for judging success, and implement systems and procedures to support the total effort of everyone
- following through – having support measures in place to ensure that projects are being taken forward and providing regular and high-quality positive and constructive feedback; when necessary, this entails ensuring that tough questions are asked and disagreements are faced and resolved constructively

- achieving results – being able to take charge and deliver high levels of performance by setting challenging goals, staying focused on the end purpose and encouraging everyone to maximise their contribution

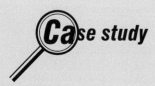

Keywords

Influencing

Is the ability to affect someone's thinking or behaviour; effective leaders are able to sway people's thinking and influence their decisions

- team playing – being able to develop positive and trusting relationships throughout the organisation, by working with people, asking their opinions, **influencing** senior management and working effectively across unit boundaries.

The value of this tool is that it is focused on behaviour and what you *do* in order to be effective. Behaviour is something that is observable; it can be described and therefore, if a person wants to, it can be changed. Generally, there are some areas where an individual feels more comfortable and confident than they do in others.

Case study

Turning good ideas into real initiatives

George was great at seeing opportunities and how the service could be improved. He would connect his ideas to relevant policy initiatives and fire people up with his enthusiasm and passion for the idea that he was championing. However, many of George's initiatives did not fulfil their early promise and potential and often gradually faded out of view. Why? George was very good at creating a vision of what could be and developing people to follow his vision. He was motivated by new and exciting ideas that required someone to lead from the front. However, he was less enthusiastic about putting in the structures and processes that were required to follow through on the ideas and turn them into sustainable, successful initiatives. This would have been all right if George had identified someone who was good at implementing a vision and following through. However, he was inclined to sell those people on his new idea, rather than let them follow through on the implementation of his previous idea.

- How would you feel working with George?
- Why might some people find George frustrating to work with?

Reflective activity

- In which of the areas of leadership activity described on page 33 do you think you are strongly active?

  Can you identify three positive examples to support that belief?

  Are there any downsides to your being strongly active in this area?

- Which of the leadership activities do you do less of?

  Is that because you are uncomfortable with those areas or because you need more knowledge and skill?

- What are the advantages of being less active in these areas? Provide three current or recent examples.

- What are the disadvantages of being less active in these areas? Provide three current or recent examples.

Kouzes and Posner (1997) have also examined effective leadership behaviours; from their research, they identified five core practices.

- **Leaders challenge the process**. They search out challenging opportunities to change, grow, innovate and improve. They take risks, and learn from the accompanying mistakes.
- **Leaders inspire a shared vision**. They envision a bright and uplifting future and engage others in shared vision by appealing to their values, intcrests, hopes and dreams.
- **Leaders enable others to act.** They promote collaboration by promoting shared goals and building trust. They strengthen people by giving power away, providing and encouraging choice, facilitating skill development, providing challenging tasks and being supportive.
- **Leaders model the way**. They set examples and role model behaviour that is consistent with shared values. They encourage the achievement of small wins, thereby promoting consistent progress and helping to build commitment.
- **Leaders encourage the heart**. They recognise individual contributions to the success of every project and regularly celebrate team accomplishments.

A third model that you are likely to come across is the Leadership Qualities Framework (LQF), which was designed with the complexities of the NHS in mind and identifies 15 leadership qualities split between 3 clusters (NHS, 2002). The LQF begins by putting personal qualities at the centre of leadership and then works outwards to 'setting the direction' and 'delivering the service', with a number of individual qualities identified within each cluster.

Table 2.5 Leadership Qualities Framework

Setting direction	Personal qualities	Delivering the service
Seizing the future	Self-belief	Leading change through people
Intellectual flexibiltiy	Self-awareness	Holding to account
Broad scanning	Self-management	Empowering others
Political astuteness	Drive for improvement	Effective and strategic influencing
Drive for results	Personal integrity	Collaborative working
(NHS, 2002)		

Evidence base

Look up additional information from www.executive.modern.nhs.uk/framework.

Equally relevant to each of the frameworks that have been discussed is the LQF's recommendation (NHS, 2002) that you have clarity of purpose – in other words, that you have thought about what it is that you are trying to achieve, and why, by using a particular framework.

Although, as you might expect, the specific language used may vary, core themes are consistent across each of the three models that we have identified; a number of these will be explored in more depth as you progress through the chapter.

Self-assessment

The above models have been thoroughly researched and validated and offer a valuable point of reference. They are 360° assessment tools and they are usually only available as part of a leadership development programme. There are several online self-assessment leadership tools; however, these have generally not been validated, which is why there is no charge. Nevertheless, these tools can still provide some useful questions to get you thinking about your current performance and future potential as a leader.

Evidence base

Look at www.turningpointprogram.org/toolkit.

In contrast, there is the more popular 'airport' literature, for example the *Fish Guide* (Charthouse Learning, 2002) and *Who Moved My Cheese?* (Johnson, 1998), which provide an insightful and motivational approach to leadership. Their purpose is to enthuse you and encourage you to take responsibility for your style and approach to work and life as a whole.

Fish (Lundin, Paul and Christensen, 1995) is an excellent book that draws on the parable of a real-life fish market to demonstrate how it is possible for ordinary people to turn around their work environment. It combines the concepts of leaderfulness and working within your circle of influence to effect change.

The authors identify four interlocking principles:

- **Play**. Create an environment where there is mutual trust and people feel able to be light-hearted.
- **Make their day**. Make a positive impact on someone's day, for example by saying 'thank you for doing that', asking if there is anything else you can do for them, or remembering that it is someone's birthday.
- **Be there**. This relates to your mindset when you are interacting with someone; give them a 100% of your attention however long the interaction is.

- **Choose your attitude**. Acknowledge that you may not be able to control some of the things that happen to you, for example traffic jams or staff sickness, but that you do have a choice about how you respond. Whether you get grumpy, blame others, moan about how awful it is, or you look at the situation, decide on the priorities and then do something about achieving them in a proactive and cheerful manner.

Reflective activity

Read through Table 2.6 and consider the interaction between the first and second columns. Then, in the third column identify examples of when, where and with whom you perhaps engage in the different mindsets of 'resentful' or 'helpful'. The examples could relate to work, family or the social environment.

Table 2.6

Who are you being? How are you feeling?	When you are?	Your example of when you are . . . .
Resentful	Cleaning back yard with a partner and grumbling	
Helpful	Cleaning back yard with a partner and making the work easier	
Manipulative	Coaching someone to make them do it 'your way'	
Supportive	Coaching someone to help them meet their goals	
Inconsiderate	Listening and having side conversations in staff meetings	
Engaged	Listening and contributing in staff meetings	
Fearful	Hearing feedback and becoming defensive	
Grateful	Hearing feedback and accepting it	
Impatient	Rushing through staff/carer/staff member interactions	
Effective	Being with the patient/carer/staff member fully during each interaction	
Living wholeheartedly		

(adapted from Charthouse Learning, 2002)

- How do the examples that you have identified help or hinder you in being an effective leader?
- Are there any recurring scenarios?
- Do any of your examples reflect the interests, abilities, values and needs that you identified in the exercise on page 24?

Leadership assessment

There are four key ways of assessing your leadership style:

- through reflection
- by inviting and being open to feedback
- by completing a self-assessment questionnaire, and
- by participating in a 360° appraisal.

360° leadership appraisals

In a 360° appraisal, you receive feedback from your boss, peers and direct reports in addition to your own perceptions of your self. Whilst that may initially feel a little scary, it is also very enlightening and helpful. After all, you will often hear people saying, for example, 'I assume I am doing an OK job; no one has said otherwise' or 'I don't understand why they reacted like that'. Both are symptoms of a lack of clarity about how people perceive and experience working with us and, although everyone identifies the importance of open communication and regular feedback, in reality we do not often receive (or give feedback) as regularly as would be helpful.

A good 360° appraisal should:

- provide feedback that is objective
- be descriptive
- avoid making judgements about whether your behaviour is good or bad
- relate to behaviour and its potential impact
- give you insight into your strengths as well as any areas for development.

The fundamental purpose of 360° feedback is developmental. It will give you an opportunity to understand how others perceive and experience your behaviours and the impact that this may have on their working relationship with you. A good 360° appraisal tool acts like a Johari window (see figure) and facilitates robust self-reflection. It should help to re-iterate those behaviours and their impact, be they strengths or weaknesses, which you already know about and that are known to others, that is, 'open' behaviours.

The appraisal should provide you with feedback on areas that others know about, but may not have fed back to you and to which, in effect, you were 'blind'. Then there are those areas that deep down you do know about but have 'hidden' by not sharing with others. However, other people experience the impact of the 'hidden' behaviour, and highlighting this behaviour through your 360° feedback may begin to explain how and why people respond to you in the way that they do. Then there are strengths, or areas for development, which remain 'unknown' until something happens that flushes them out into the open.

	Known to self	Not known
Known to others	Open	Blind
Not known to others	Hidden	Unknown

The Johari window (adapted from Luft and Ingham, 1995)

There are several models and frameworks (Schon, 1983; Johns, 2004) to choose from to help guide the process of reflection, and, as a health care professional, you will have been introduced to many during the course of your training and work career.

An important starting point for these models is being aware of the questions that you ask yourself and how these can direct your thinking. Adams (2004) describes how the questions we ask ourselves can take us down a learner (constructive and empowering) path or a judger (negative and blaming) path.

Reflective activity

- When did you last use a learner path question?
- How did it help the situation?
- With hindsight, identify a work-related situation when you could have used a learner path question but did not do so.
- Now consider and identify how using a learner path question could have improved the outcome.

Table 2.7 Examples of judger/learner path questions

Judger path questions	Learner path questions
What went wrong?	What happened? What's useful here to know more about? What do I want to learn?
Who's to blame?	What am I responsible for?
How can I prove I'm right?	What are the facts?
How can I protect myself?	What is the big picture?
What is wrong with me?	What can I learn from this?
What's wrong with them? Why are they so stupid?	What is happening for the other person? How are they thinking and feeling?
Why am I no good at this?	What could I do? What are my choices? What's best to do now?
Why bother?	What's possible?
Outcomes	*Outcomes*
Automatic reactions Blame focused Win–lose and lose–win relationships	Thoughtful choices Solution focused Win–win relationships
Impact on you and others	*Impact on you and others*
Undermined Anger Loss of confidence	Empowered Energised Increased knowledge/skill/attitude

(adapted from Adams, 2004)

What impression do you generate as a leader?

An additional component of effective, modern leadership is awareness of the impression that you make on people: first impressions and lasting impressions. This is important because part of your leadership role depends not just on how you present yourself and behave within your immediate team, but also on how you contribute to other people's perception and experience of the team, department or organisation within which you are working.

Whilst many of the behaviours that we have described so far, such as integrity, motivation, strong communication skills, and so on, are part of the lasting perception that people will have of you, it is also important to pay attention to the initial impact that you have on people. Everett (2005) suggests that we ask ourselves the following four questions:

- How do I come across when I meet people for the first time?
- What image do I project?
- What three words would people use to describe me?
- Which one behavioural or image trait might be worth changing?

A useful additional question to ask yourself is, 'Would the answers to the above questions be different according to whether the other person was a patient, a senior manager, a patient advocate, a consultant, a health care assistant, and so on?' If so, why and what impact might that have?

Leading yourself/leading others

The lens through which you view the world, or particular people or incidents, and how you then filter that view will have an impact on your thinking and therefore your behaviour and, in turn, the events around you.

Reflective activity

You want to discuss best practice as regards to oral hygiene care with a mature health care assistant with several years' experience, as you believe that her practice is not up to date.

Take a few minutes to think about and make some notes in answer to the following questions:

- How would you feel about discussing the issues? (not worried, justified, confident, nervous, wary?)

- What are your lenses and filters with regard to this issue? (You might have been brought up to believe that you should not question your elders. You may have previous experience of doing something similar and it went well, or perhaps it went badly and you were shouted at or mocked for questioning.)

- How do your answers to the above two questions then impact on your behaviour? (You might be blasé and rush in and make a mess of it. You may have done something similar before, which went well, and so you feel confident about approaching the situation. Alternatively, you might feel nervous or wary and not have a positive experience to draw upon. Would that stop you addressing the issue or result in your putting off dealing with it for so long that the situation becomes even more difficult?)

Leading innovation

Health care delivery is constantly changing. It always has and will continue to do so: in part because of clinical developments and in part because of wider demographic changes and policy changes at a political level.

The leader of today and tomorrow needs to be able not just to embrace and respond positively to change but also to be able to initiate it by exploring how else things could be done to improve the quality and efficiency of health care. Not only do you need to be able to see possibilities and then have the energy and passion to take them forward, but you also have to have the skills to influence and persuade in order to get your ideas and those of the people around you put into action.

Increasing reference is being made by the Department of Health (1998, 1999, 2001) within policy documents and within the wider health care literature (Plsek and Greenhalgh, 2001) to the perceived need for people working in health care to demonstrate more **flexibility** in how they approach their work. The underpinning belief is that the more creative and innovative strategies that individuals are able to draw upon and use within their daily practice, the more responsive they are to the challenges of leading and delivering effective health care services and the better able they are to respond.

> Nurses who provide care in an innovative and creative manner are highly valued by both professionals and patients.
>
> Ferguson (1992)

Being creative with patients and carers is rarely a problem for health care professionals. They will be very resourceful when it comes to engaging with a patient to complete their physiotherapy exercises, drink enough fluid or generally implement an aspect of their care plan. However, often when it comes to working with other staff members, characteristics such as persistence, resourcefulness and creativity do not seem to transfer. Instead, what you will hear is a range of killer phrases that instantly lock up people's creativity.

Mental locks

The following are examples of responses that act as mental locks:

- **The right answer**. That will work; that must be the right answer to this situation; we don't need to look any further. In reality, for most leadership decisions, there is no right answer, just a number of potentially good options. The challenge is to generate four or five options and choose the best, rather than go with the first one that you think of.
- **That's not logical**. I don't understand what you are saying; you cannot explain clearly how it is going to work, so I don't think it has any value.
- **Follow the rules**. We should be following procedure, and I am not comfortable doing something different to the usual way.
- **Be practical**. That is all very creative, but we need something sensible that we can do now (I can't see how your idea could be adapted or translated into a viable option).
- **We don't have time**. I know your idea may have some value, but either I don't feel comfortable with it or I want a quick fix (I know time invested up front saves time in the long run, but . . .).

⊶🔑 *Keywords*

Flexibility

Is the ability to change or respond to different circumstances in different ways, using different strategies. This is more than just learning a set of behaviours. Your challenge is developing and then sustaining both a mindset and a skill set that will enable you to be flexible

- **That's not my area.** I am hiding behind either not being expert in that area or not having responsibility for it and so, maybe because I don't want to look foolish, avoid offering an outsider's opinion.
- **Don't be foolish**. It seems obvious to me, but I don't want to be laughed at or ridiculed for saying something that may be too simple or misses some point that I don't know about.
- **To err is wrong**. I cannot afford to make a mistake or fail; I might get shouted at or feel foolish. I must always make the right decision and be successful with any new idea or initiative.
- **I'm not creative**. I'm no good at drawing or arty things. In leadership, creativity is about seeing possibilities, new solutions or a different way of doing something and not artistic ability.

(adapted from Von Oech, 1992)

You may also have your own phrases that have become established in your vocabulary, providing a 'get-out' clause so that you do not have to engage in creativity yourself or be open and receptive to other people's creativity. Some of these will be long-held beliefs or perceptions that are now holding you back.

Reflective activity

- Which of the mental locks described above (or something similar) do you use or at least think?
- Identify two occasions when you have used a mental lock. What was the impact?
- What could you do to 'disable' one of your mental locks?
- What mental locks are you on the receiving end of and how do they leave you feeling?

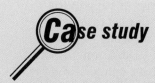 **se study**

The impact of assumptions

Danielle had transferred from radiography to theatres. In a staff meeting a few weeks after she had transferred, there was a big discussion around yet another complaint that theatres had received regarding the movement of patients between the theatres and the ward. After listening for five minutes or so, Danielle spoke up and began to say that when she had worked in the radiography department they had also had similar complaints but, after a number of attempts, had successfully resolved the situation. Without waiting to hear how the situation had been resolved, one person said very loudly, 'Look, radiography is quite different to theatres. When you have been with us a bit longer, you will realise that there is no hope of whatever it was working for us.' Danielle went quiet and it was another three months before her experience was listened to in a non-related conversation over a coffee and adopted with the same positive impact that had been experienced in radiography.

continued

- How else could Danielle have responded during the original meeting in order to share her experience and learning?
- What responsibility did the rest of the staff present in the meeting have:
  - to help Danielle be listened to?
  - to address the behaviour of the member of staff who had 'silenced' Danielle?
- What impact do you think the incident might have had on Danielle's contribution to the team?

Danielle was not being particularly whacky or creative: she was simply relating an experience in one environment to another and seeing what might usefully transfer. The stumbling block was someone else's very large mental lock.

Key points **Top tips**

For those of you who are still struggling with your inner self and believe that you are not creative, the good news is that research studies show us three things:

- Creativity is an inherent ability that we all have (Zelenko, 1993).
- It is more developed in some than in others (Ferguson, 1992).
- It is a skill that can be learnt and refined (McConathy, 1990).

There is a plethora of tools and techniques to help you be more creative in how you think, generate ideas, problem solve and make decisions. People such as Tony Buzan (1993) and Edward de Bono (1992) have written extensively about creativity and have produced a number of easy-to-use resources. Similarly, there are many websites providing a range of useful techniques and exercises.

Influencing and whole brain leadership

Influencing is a key facet of leadership, whether to inspire people with your vision or motivate them to give you some money or support the implementation of relevant structures to enable your idea to get off the ground. Effective leaders have the ability to affect someone's opinions, actions and behaviour. They appreciate that we all process and respond to information differently and therefore present ideas, opinions and information in a variety of ways in order to persuade people of their value. Whilst creativity and innovation are clearly important aspects of this, and there is a need to develop people's abilities in these areas, it is important that they are not valued to the detriment of those other leadership behaviours that help to turn good ideas into sustainable realities. Unlike many frameworks, the Whole Brain Model (Herrmann, 1993) takes a holistic approach to looking at your thinking preferences and the impact that these have on everything that you do. The model provides an easy-to-use framework for anyone wanting to be a more effective leader.

The more flexible you are – in other words, the more you use your whole brain, as opposed to just the left-hand side (LHS) or the right-hand side (RHS) – the more likely you are to influence a greater number of people. Equally, the less flexible you are, the more difficult it will be to engage a cross section of people as opposed to those that you always manage to engage. So, if you hear yourself saying 'Am I talking to a brick wall?' ask yourself 'Am I saying the same thing to everyone and only appear to be engaging a few?' Would you use the same PowerPoint presentation for the community rehabilitation team as you would for the executive team of the organisation? Hopefully, you have answered no because you recognise that they will be influenced by different arguments. The same principle applies within the rehabilitation team itself. Members of staff will be influenced to different degrees by different factors, and your challenge is to address all of those factors within one presentation in order to maximise your chances of being heard by everyone as opposed to the proverbial brick wall.

The Whole Brain Model (Herrmann, 1993) has grown out of hard science; creative and innovative approaches to learning and communicating have resulted in a well-researched and validated model that produces a profile of a person's thinking preferences in relation to four specific quadrants or preference types.

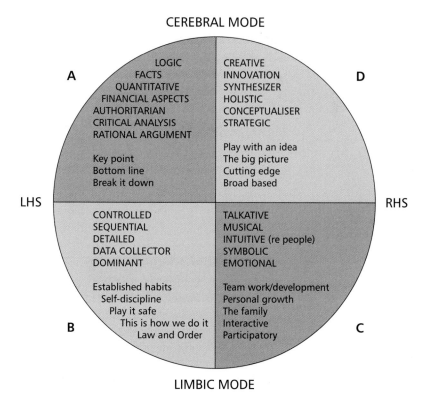

The brain's thinking preferences (adapted from Herrmann, 1993)

People vary as regards to how comfortable they are working in any one or more of the quadrants. The more flexible you can be, and the more quadrants you can comfortably operate in, the more people you are likely to be able to connect with, and work with, which can only help your effectiveness as a leader. If, for example, you want to influence someone who has a strong quadrant A or AB preference, you need to think about presenting a factual, logical argument and providing examples and evidence to support your case.

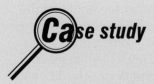

Understanding each other's thinking preferences

Sam was very good at making sure that there were systems and processes in place to ensure the smooth running of the working day. For most routine situations, there were clear guidelines and structures and everyone knew what should happen. A decision was taken to close the old hospital and both to re-structure and to re-locate the service into a new community hospital. For some, this was a great opportunity to deliver the service differently and introduce new technologies and ways of working to provide patients with a new and more patient-focused service. Sam, however, found such discussions very difficult as it was not exactly clear how some of these new initiatives would work in reality. Other team members felt that as long as the principles and patient safety were right, they could work on the 'how' as the new service evolved, and then Sam could do what he was good at, which was to make things appear 'routine'.

- Using the figure on page 45 as a reference point, in which quadrant(s) would you position:
  (a) Sam
  (b) the other team members?
- What do you think people in quadrant B find difficult about working with people in quadrant D and vice versa?
- What might be the benefit to each group of working with people who have a preference for a different quadrant?
- In which of the quadrants are you most comfortable?
- Are there any quadrants that you dislike? What is the impact of that?
- Identify a current initiative where you are trying to engage people and persuade them to 'go with you' on the initiative that you are proposing (this can be a small or large initiative). Design a presentation that will have an impact in relation to all four quadrants and therefore maximise the likelihood of your engaging those people.

Developmental options

So what can you do if you want to work actively to increase your effectiveness as a leader? You can decide to invest in yourself and undertake some self-managed development. This involves your taking responsibility for identifying and directing your own development.

Having worked through this chapter, completed the exercises and reflected on the case studies, what more can you do if you want to take action to increase your effectiveness as a leader? The following table contains a range of activities that you could choose to do. It specifically does not include attending a leadership development programme as, although that might be relevant, it may also have financial implications. The options identified are all generally 'free'. The list is not exhaustive, and, if you identify something different that would suit your needs, you should build it into your action plan.

Table 2.8 Development options

Activity	Action Steps
Extend your scope of practice	Ask if work can be delegated to you
Project working – volunteer	Offer to be part of a working group that is being set up. Volunteer for something that will increase your knowledge, skill and networks
Work shadowing	Be clear about your purpose, what is it that you are aiming to learn and who would be the best person to shadow to help achieve that aim
Secondments	Step outside your comfort zone and take on a role or project that will result in your being seconded for a period of time
Job rotation	Broaden your horizons, volunteer to be part of a job-rotation scheme or introduce the idea into your work environment
Training in specific skills: e.g. presentation skills	Observe someone you think is good at the skill. Read a key text for practical tips. Ask someone to be a critical friend, providing you with honest feedback on your performance while you are developing the skill
Find an appropriate mentor	Be clear about what you are looking for from a mentor and the style of mentorship you are looking for. Be bold and think *big*
Become a mentor for someone else	Be clear about what they are looking for from a mentor and what you can offer. Read a key text and be clear about the underpinning principles
Form/join an action learning set	Seek some like-minded people who are looking to develop their skills and understanding of the wider picture
Tap into new networks	Join a new professional interest group, attend an open meeting, workshop or seminar that will include people you don't usually meet. Think what you can bring to the network as well as what you might gain
Read	Make a top 5–10 list and commit to reading the items on the list
Websites	Bookmark six websites in your favourites file and visit them once a month
Undertake some research	Offer to support someone undertaking some research or identify something that needs to be further understood and explore it
Do some writing	Write about something about which you feel passionate
Seek feedback	Be clear about what you are seeking feedback on and why, and that the timing is appropriate
Keep a learning diary/log	Difficult to sustain so requires discipline to get into and keep the habit
Visit other comparable workplaces	Arrange visits, invite people to visit you and jointly benchmark your work against similar areas
Attend meetings organised by your local professional body	Be an active member of a professional body, access information and contribute to the discussions and debates (Zelenko, 1993)
Write a personal development plan (PDP)	A good PDP should be challenging but realistic, written in specific and measurable language and goals and shared with someone else – you are more likely to implement your PDP if you commit to someone else

The future direction of leadership

The publication of *Commissioning a Patient Led NHS* (Department of Health, 2005) and the White Paper *Our Health, Our Care, Our Say* (Department of Health, 2006) definitely signal some significant proposed changes in the type of working environment that health care professionals might encounter during the next decade.

To date, the choices with regard to where you might work have centred on either private, charitable, or public (state) health care provision, followed by either inpatient services or community-based services. Over the next 10 years, the provision of health care by social enterprises is set to increase significantly. The Department of Health has indicated its intentions to promote and support this type of health care provision through the establishment of the Social Enterprise Unit (www.dh.gov.uk).

Just as the understanding of the nature of leadership has changed significantly during the last century, so too is the type of health care organisation and employment environment in which you will be working set to alter quite dramatically during the present century. This will, in turn, have an impact on the type of leadership behaviours that you will need to demonstrate in order to be effective. You have explored the importance of the leader as a creator and innovator; being an intrapreneur, who helps to generate ideas and solutions and is open to doing things differently, is a requirement not an 'add-on'. The next decade will take those behaviours a step further forward and place them within a social enterprise working environment.

Conclusion

Your effectiveness as a leader will be judged by everything you say and do. Your challenge is to be sufficiently self-aware to understand how you are perceived by others and then to be open, receptive and responsive to feedback both with regard to your areas of strength and to any areas for development. This should be a continuous process, not a one-off activity.

How you behave and therefore how you are perceived as a leader is your choice. A useful strategy is to think in metaphors, as that will free you up to think more conceptually and to generate a big picture of how you want to be as a leader.

Reflective activity

If you were to represent your approach to leadership as if it was a car, what would it be?

Take five minutes to draw or write down what the car would look like. Would it be a saloon, a vintage, a 4 x 4, or a racing car? Would it have a large engine, any luggage space, run on petrol or diesel? What sort of headlights would it have? What would be the colour and design of its paintwork? Would it be a two-door or a four-door model? Be as detailed as you can be as the more specific your description, the clearer the picture you will generate of your approach to leadership.

Having drawn or created a written description of your leadership style as a car, now ask yourself:

- Is your car fit for purpose?
- Does it need servicing or upgrading?
- When might you need to change this car?
- What would the new car look like and why?

Rapid recap

Check your progress so far by working through each of the following questions.

1. Describe the difference between position power and personal power.
2. Name five mental locks that people use that inhibit their creative ability.
3. How could you use the Whole Brain Model to help you at work?
4. Why might 'learner' questions enable you to move a situation forward further than if you were using 'judger' questions?
5. Identify the four key words of the Fish philosophy and describe how you could make them relevant to your world.
6. Identify five developmental activities that you could include in a personal development plan.

If you have difficulty with more than one of the questions, read through the section again to refresh your understanding before moving on.

References

Adams, M. (2004) *Change Your Questions, Change Your Life: 7 Powerful Tools for Life and Work*. Berrett-Koehler Publishers Inc., San Fransisco.

Buzan, T. (1993) *The Mind Map Book*. BBC Books, London.

Charthouse Learning (2002) *Fish Guide – A Remarkable Way to Boost Morale and Improve Results*. Coronet Books, Philadelphia.

Cunningham, G. and Kitson, A. (2000) An Evaluation of The RCN Clinical Leadership Development Programme: Parts 1 and 2. *Nursing Standard*, **15**(12): 34–40.

De Bono, E. (1992) *Serious Creativity*. Harper Collins Publishing, New York.

Department of Health (1998) *Improving Working Lives*. Department of Health, London.

Department of Health (1999) *Making a Difference – Strengthening the Contribution of Nursing, Midwifery and Health Visiting Contribution to Health and Health Care*. Department of Health, London.

Department of Health (2001) *Shifting the Balance of Power within the NHS: Securing Delivery*. Department of Health, London.

Department of Health (2005) *Commissioning a Patient Led NHS*. The Stationery Office, London.

Department of Health (2006) *Our Health, Our Care, Our Say*. The Stationery Office, London.

Everett, L. (2005) Taking Control of Your Personal Brand. *Training Journal*, (Feb.): 26–28.

Farmer, B. (1993) The Use and Abuse of Power in Nursing. *Nursing Standard*, **7**(24 Feb.): 33–36.

Ferguson, L. (1992) Teaching for Creativity. *Nurse Educator*, **17**(1): 9–16.

French, J.R.P. and Raven, B. (1968) The Bases of Social Power. In: *Group Dynamics Research and Theory*, 3rd edn. (ed. Cartwright, D and Zander, A.F.). Harper & Row, New York.

Goleman, D. (1998) What Makes a Leader? *Harvard Business Review*. (Nov–Dec.): 93–102.

Handy, C. (1993) *Understanding Organisations*. Penguin Group, London.

Herrmann, N. (1993) *The Creative Brain*. The Ned Herrmann Group, North Carolina.

Johns, C. (2004) *Becoming a Reflective Practitioner,* 2nd edn. Blackwell Publishing, Oxford.

Johnson, S. (1998) *Who Moved My Cheese?* Vermilion, London.

Kouzes, J. and Posner, B. (1997) *Leadership Practices Inventory,* 2nd edn. – Participant's Workbook. Josey-Bass Pfeiffer, California.

Kreitner, R. (1995) *Management*. Houghton Mifflin, Boston.

Lundin, S., Paul, H. and Christensen, J. (1995) *Fish – A Remarkable Way to Boost Moral and Improve Results*. Hodder & Stoughton, London.

Luft, J. and Ingham, H. (1955) The Johari Window: A Graphic Model of Interpersonal Awareness. *Proceedings of the Western Training Laboratory in Group Development*. UCLA, Los Angeles.

Management Research Group (1992) *Leadership Effectiveness Analysis*. Management Research Group, Munich.

Marquis, B. and Huston, C. (2003) *Leadership Roles and Management Functions in Nursing Theory and Application*, 5th edn. Lippincott, Williams and Wilkins, Philadelphia.

McConathy, D. (1990). Theories of Creativity. *Journal of Bio-Communication*, **17**(2): 5–11.

McLean, J.W. and Weitzel, W. (1992) *Leadership – Magic, Myth or Method?* American Management Association, New York.

NHS (2002) *The Leadership Qualities Framework*. The Stationery Office, London.

Oxford University Press (2001) *Oxford Dictionary, Thesaurus and Wordpower Guide*. Oxford University Press, Oxford.

Plsek, P. and Greenhalgh, T. (2001) The Challenge of Complexity in Health Care. *BMJ*, **323**(15 Sep.): 625–628.

Raelin, J. (2003) *Creating Leaderful Organisations: How to Bring Out the Leadership in Everyone*. Berrett-Koehler Publishers Inc., San Fransisco.

Salvage, J. (1999) Speaking out . . . supersisters . . . clinical leadership. *Nursing Times*, **95**(21): 22.

Schon, D. (1983) *The Reflective Practitioner*. Avebury Press, Aldershot.

Smith, S. (1997) The Loneliness of a Long-term Leader. *Nursing Times*, **93**(12): 30–32.

Stodgill, R.M. (1974) *Handbook of Leadership*. Free Press, New York.

Van Oech, R. (1992) *A Whack on The Side of The Head – How You Can Be More Creative*. Creative Think, California.

Zelenko, T. (1993). Creative thinking: One of the factors to increase creative potential of students of technical higher education institutions. *New Era in Education*, **74**(2): 51.

Useful websites

www.businessballs.com/johariwindowmodel.htm

Centre for Creative Leadership: www.ccl.org

Centre for Leadership Studies: www.leadership-studies.com

Harvard Business Review: www.hbr.org

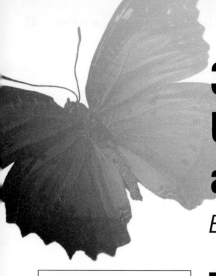

3
Understanding yourself as a manager

Elaine McNichol

Learning outcomes

By the end of this chapter you should be able to:

★ Describe and discuss the different theories of management

★ Discuss the relationship and balance between leadership and management

★ Identify and discuss the relevance of essential management behaviours

★ Understand the balance between responsibility, authority and accountability

★ Assess your own understanding of key management skills

★ Describe and discuss a range of developmental options in relation to management.

Introduction

You could be forgiven for thinking that management was leadership's poor relation. Whilst we have had national leadership programmes, there has been no such emphasis in recent years with regard to the development of management skills. Yet, strong, robust management skills are an essential part of the professional's toolkit.

Leadership and management are a natural partnership. The skill is getting the balance between them right.

In brief, leadership constitutes seeing and setting the vision for where you, the team and patient care are going; effective management will then help you to put together the plan for how to get there, by when, with who doing what and with what resources.

This chapter will explore the key aspects of understanding yourself as a manager and identify a number of practical models and strategies that you can apply.

Management

We all have a management responsibility. Whatever our position, this begins with an individual responsibility to manage ourselves appropriately. As a student professional, this starts in relation to the management of your contribution to patient care and the management of your interactions and relationships with other members of the immediate team and with other teams that are part

Leadership and management in balance

Leadership ⚖ Management

of the wider context. As your career progresses, so the shape and form of your management responsibility changes in accordance with the changing nature and demands of your role.

The skill is in knowing when to lead and when to manage. This is summed up by Covey (1989), who states that:

> effectiveness – often even survival – does not depend solely on how much effort we expend, but whether or not the effort we expend is in the right place.
>
> Covey (1989, p. 101)

In other words, we can put a lot of effort into managing situations, but, unless there is a clear vision, of where managing these situations will help take us to, we might be putting our energies into the wrong activity.

It is no good working out the best route to get to Dover and dealing with all the traffic problems on the way, if we have missed the fact that the destination has changed and we are supposed to be going to York. This is particularly relevant in the fast-changing world of health care policy and practice. Whilst the destination should always be 'best patient care', the context is continually shifting. In order to 'manage' the delivery of 'best patient care', you will always need to be looking to the future and at whether the context is changing.

Management and leadership are part of the same continuum and the ratio of management to leadership is determined by the needs of the situation.

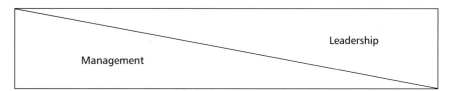

Management/leadership continuum

If you have been asked to 'sort an issue out' and ensure that minimum standards and safety requirements are met, then the ability to assess the situation, allocate priorities to what needs to be done, delegate the tasks appropriately and ensure that they are completed to the required standard are all essential. It will also be necessary for you to recognise the level of authority that you have to undertake the task and to be willing to use the position power that you have to get the job done (see Table 3.3, p. 62). It is likely that you will be using behaviours and approaches that have a strong management focus.

If, however, you have been asked to develop some good practice guidelines and minimum standards for a new service that is being developed, then you are more likely to canvas opinion, review what is happening elsewhere, explore the underpinning principles and philosophy of the new service, draft guidelines and seek feedback from those who will be implementing them. In other words, your approach will be at the leadership end of the continuum.

A key factor that will influence your approach to a particular situation is 'time'. Management is often about here-and-now issues that need dealing with promptly, whereas leadership is often associated more with equally important but less immediate decision making. This can result in crisis management, and we will explore this point further in the section on time management (see p. 58).

Theories and models

As with leadership, a body of knowledge and a number of perspectives in relation to management have emerged over the years, reflecting the cultural and philosophical changes of the era. As these can be found in numerous well-established management textbooks, they will not be repeated here. Instead, this chapter will focus on three specific theories that reflect different philosophical approaches to management and may therefore be captured in your reflections in the last exercise on page 78. Table 3.1 will provide you with a brief summary.

Reflective activity

- Which of the theories outlined in Table 3.1 do you believe best reflects your perceptions and beliefs regarding management?
- What is the implication of that in relation to how you respond to people managing you?
- How do your perceptions and beliefs influence your approach to management?

These are quite fundamental questions and, as you work through both this chapter and the book as a whole, you may find that you want to re-visit these questions and adapt your responses as your thinking develops.

You as a manager of relationships

This section is first and foremost about how you manage yourself, then how you manage situations and your relationships with those around you. It is likely that many of the 'issues' that you encounter during a working day arise from relationships in the workplace. Your overall effectiveness as a health care professional rests on your ability to build successful relationships with people at all levels both within and outside

Table 3.1 Theories and models of management

Theory	Characteristics	Implications
Taylor – Scientific management	About adopting a systematic approach to finding the best way of completing the task. Jobs are scientifically broken down into their component parts, with specific instructions on how best to complete them in order to maximise productivity. This is a mechanistic approach to the job in hand and the backdrop to concepts such as 'payment by results' and 'management by exception'	There is a clear division of work. The focus is entirely on the task to be completed. The risk is that if a worker is only seeing one part of the picture, they can not only get bored but also fail to appreciate the wider consequences of their action or non-action for the whole job. Also, for some people, the 'best' method may be different because of their own idiosyncrasies
McGregor – Theory X and Theory Y	Theory X assumes that people dislike work and are there because they have to be and must therefore be controlled, directed and coerced to ensure that organisational goals are met. The belief is that most workers prefer to be directed and have no or minimal responsibility	Managers do the planning and take the decisions; they supervise closely and tend to motivate workers by making it clear that there will be positive or negative consequences of doing or not doing something that the workers are told to do
	Theory Y assumes that people are happy to be at work and that they have their own self-direction and control and motivation to get the job done. The emphasis is on meeting both the needs of the job and the goals of the worker. If successful, the worker is happy to take on responsibility and to engage proactively and creatively with their role	The manager involves others in decision making, is happy to delegate, monitors at a distance and motivates staff through rewards such as praise and recognition
Human relations	Builds upon Theory Y principles and believes that work satisfies a complex range of needs for the individual that extend beyond 'how much money they earn'. Work is viewed as a social microcosm where the culture, values and norms are important for the wellbeing of the individual and, therefore, their ability to perform	The manager needs to take time to know what is important to individual staff within the context of work in order to know how best to reward and motivate them. Requires time and personal commitment from the manager. Some would say that there is a risk that the balance between the needs of the individual and the needs of the organisation has become skewed

the organisation. In addition, the quality of human relationships in the workplace is recognised as having a direct impact on people's job satisfaction and their satisfaction with their lives overall (Judge and Watanabe, 1993). In order to understand others, you first need to understand yourself.

As discussed in Chapter 2, the purpose of greater self-understanding is to help you work better with other people, be they patients, colleagues or the public. Self-understanding supports personal growth and development and contributes to improved relationships. The awareness and insight that you gain provides you with choices. It enables you to press the PAUSE button, think and then decide on the best response. This is important because much of our daily contact with people operates on a reactive level.

⸿elɟɘЯ *Reflective activity*

Think about who or what you react to.

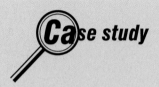

Poor patient care?

A practice nurse is working in a GP surgery; yesterday, Dr. Jones reprimanded her about an aspect of poor patient care that he believed had resulted from her practice. She went home feeling quite angry about how he had addressed the situation with her; she felt that he was looking for someone to blame.

Today, Dr. Jones came into the clinic room where she was and said, 'Why has Mr. Barrett's blood test not been done?'

- If you were the practice nurse, what would be your first reaction?
- What would be your second reaction?

Now imagine that the practice nurse had been pre-warned by a colleague that Dr. Jones was looking for her to ask why Mr. Barrett's blood test has not been done.

If you were the practice nurse, what would your response be now, when Dr. Jones found you and asked the question?

Your second reaction may have been the same as your first; however, being pre-warned has given you some time to think (press the PAUSE button) and consider the question in a more rounded way. Maybe no one asked you to do the blood test. Maybe someone else was asked to do it. Maybe you have taken the blood and sent it off for testing and the results have not yet come back, or have not yet been filed in the patient's notes, or have been lost. The likelihood is that, with time to think, you moved beyond some of the anger from yesterday, thought through a number of possible reasons for the missing blood test results and were able to respond in a professional manner when Dr. Jones asked you the question.

The key issue here is that a reaction is a knee-jerk behaviour, with very little if any thought, whereas a response means that you had a choice: you could do or say at least one of two things.

In times of danger, knee-jerk reactions serve us very well and are likely to help save our lives. However, we are rarely in situations of danger at work (although it might feel like you are under fire sometimes), and therefore an 'automatic' reaction is often not the best way of addressing a situation.

Very often our response is the reply, question or course of action that you think of on the way home. It is often with hindsight and away from the heat of the moment that you can think of the strategy that would have been a more appropriate and effective way of dealing with the situation at the time that it occurred.

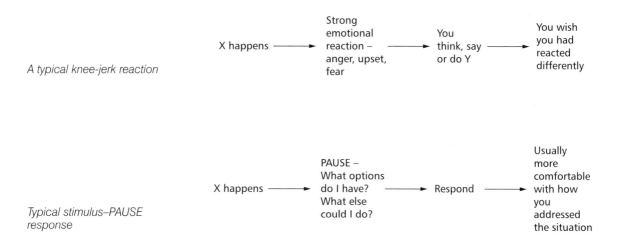

A typical knee-jerk reaction

Typical stimulus–PAUSE response

Reflective activity

Think of a situation where you have reacted and where, with hindsight, it would have been helpful if you had done something else. Make some notes about the key features of the situation.

What was the trigger for your reaction? – It might have been the tone of voice, the words the person used, a feeling of unfairness or that one of your core values was being crossed. You might not even really know. If the latter is the case, it becomes very difficult to address because you do not recognise the cause, and this is where the case for self-reflection and increasing your level of self-awareness becomes very powerful.

Many of our reactions are learnt patterns of thinking and behaving that turn into knee-jerk reactions. The purpose of increasing your self-awareness is so that you become aware of such patterns and can give yourself the choice of being able to press the PAUSE button to create some time to think before responding.

Reflective activity

Take 30 minutes and work through the questions in Table 3.2. This is a time to be honest with yourself and to consider each of the questions equally. Our behaviours have an impact on ourselves and on other people, and it is essential that you move beyond your initial thoughts to consider the longer-term consequences for yourself and others.

Table 3.2 Reactions and their consequences

What upsets you, irritates you, or makes you mad?	What is the impact?	Could you choose not to be irritated by it? How could you reframe this so that you could manage yourself more effectively?
How do you react when you are upset, irritated or mad?	What is the impact?	How else could you respond?
What are the consequences for yourself of these reactions?	What are the consequences for others of these reactions?	With which consequences are you unhappy and which would you like to change? How could you make those changes?
How do you feel afterwards?	How do other people feel afterwards?	Which feelings are you unhappy about and which would you like to change? How could you make those changes?

Are there any recurring themes or patterns? If there are, learning how to manage yourself in relation to them will give you more choices and enable you to be more effective as a health care professional.

Whilst the questions in Table 3.2 did not specifically prompt you to think about the patient, the purpose of the exercise was to highlight the importance of being aware of your knee-jerk reactions; directly or indirectly, these will be having an impact on patient care.

When answering the questions in the table, you may well have recognised that your reactions and responses could also map onto the reflective activity that you completed in the previous chapter (p. 39) in relation to judger and learner thinking and questions (Adams 2004).

Time management

An important aspect of management is ensuring that the 'right things get done the right way at the right time by the right people' (Blanchard

Keywords

Care-taker

Is someone who does things for other people that they are quite capable of doing themselves

Rescuer

Is someone who bails people out of difficult situations as opposed to holding on to the safety line and ensuring that they stay afloat whilst they work their way to safety

et al., 1994, p. 60). In reality, this is quite difficult to achieve and very often people, in trying to be supportive, find themselves acting as either **care-taker** or **rescuer**.

Someone may take on the role of care-taker for any number of reasons; perhaps there is a desire to help other people out or to be liked. However, the core component is that the care-taker has chosen to take on the role, generally because it fulfils a need in them.

Taking on the role of rescuer is also voluntary: perhaps the rescuer is uncomfortable seeing people in difficulty or they accept the role when someone shouts 'help', because, for the rescuer, it is quicker or easier than helping the person in need to stay afloat and work their way through the situation.

Clinical Caseload . . .

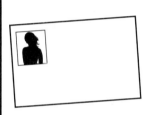

A final-year student comes to you and describes a difficulty that they are having working alongside a member of staff and asks if you will speak to the person concerned. You recognise the difficulty being described and that it will not be an easy one for the student to address, so you say, 'Leave it with me. I will follow it up.' The student came to you concerned and has left re-assured that you will deal with the problem.

- What do you think the student gained from that interaction?
- What do you think might be the implications for you as the member of staff who has said that they will follow up on the situation?

Clinical Caseload . . .

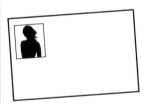

A final-year student comes to you and describes a difficulty that they are having working alongside a member of staff and asks if you will speak to the person concerned. You recognise the difficulty being described and that it will not be an easy one for the student to address. You ask the student for their thoughts about what else they could do; you coach them through the different options that they raise and agree a time when you will meet up with them and review how they managed the situation.

- What do you think the student gained from that interaction?
- What do you think might be the implications for you as the member of staff who has said that they will follow up on the situation?

Blanchard *et al.* (1994) would say that, in the first scenario, you took the student's problem (monkey) and made it your own and that as a result you have compromised both of you. Not only has the student become more dependent on you, but also the process is likely to erode their self-esteem and confidence further and they are now more likely to come to you with 'issues'. As a result of either care-taking or rescuing them, you have not only unnecessarily added to your own workload, but quite probably inappropriately taken on an issue that you will not be able to resolve, as it is between two other people and you were not directly involved.

A key facet of managing your time effectively is how you manage the issues that people bring to you. In particular, you need to recognise when it is appropriate for you to intervene. In the second scenario, you enabled the student to 'park' the monkey, in effect take the weight off their shoulders, whilst they talked the issue through with you. You built up their confidence by engaging them actively in identifying possible next steps and then helped to coach them through these.

So how do you keep the monkey on the right back?

There are a range of strategies that you can use:

- Have a toy monkey on your desk or a picture of a monkey on your wall or locker door as a visual reminder. This works on two levels: first, other people will ask you, 'Why have you got a picture of a monkey on your wall?' Each time you answer, you have an opportunity to explain the principle to more people, increasing the likelihood of them changing their behaviour, understanding any changes in your behaviour and also the rational behind those changes. In addition, the more you explain why, the more likely you are to implement the principles. There is a strong psychological adage that 'We believe what we hear ourselves say'. Therefore, the more you talk about the principles of 'keeping the monkey on the right back', the more likely you are to adhere to them.

- Secondly, having a visible, visual reminder, as described above, is hard to ignore and you are therefore more likely to change your behaviours.

- Press the PAUSE button – when someone approaches you about an 'issue' to which they want an answer, resist the inclination to deal with it there and then – unless it is a clinical priority. Instead, ask if you can talk to them about it when you have got some spare time and then give them a specific time when that can happen, for example '3.00 p.m. today or 9.00 a.m. tomorrow'. Similarly, when you want an answer to an 'issue', press the PAUSE button and ask yourself whether an answer is needed there and then or if you would be better booking a time to discuss the issue with the person concerned.

- Re-frame your thinking – if, in taking on or solving people's 'issues', your intent is to be helpful, then you are actually doing the opposite. By taking on the issue, you are depriving them of the learning and experience that they will gain by working through the situation.

Responsibility, authority and accountability

Effective managers take the responsibility that goes with their roles, use the authority that is aligned with their positions and demonstrate accountability for their actions. This is an area where to be an effective manager you need to demonstrate that your actions match your words.

Responsibility, authority and accountability are like the three legs of a stool. If any of the legs is out of synch, there is a risk that your stool might start to wobble and you will begin to feel an imbalance and the stress that comes with that.

Being effective is being both clear and proactive with regard to these three areas.

Responsibility

This is usually attached to the position that you hold and is about what is yours to own. 'You are responsible for . . .'

Responsibility is something that should be both given and, very importantly, accepted. It is not uncommon to hear a manager say that they have given someone responsibility for doing something, yet the individual concerned is either unaware that they have been given the responsibility or is unclear about how to carry out the responsibility but has not felt able to say so.

With responsibility comes obligation (Marriner-Tomey, 1996, p. 69). By accepting the responsibility, you also accept the obligation to do whatever is required to fulfil the task and the obligation associated with it.

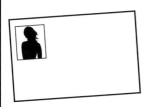

Clinical Caseload . . .

A member of staff has phoned in sick and you are asked if you will take responsibility for contacting all the patients that are due to see the sick member of staff and rearrange their appointments. If you say yes, then the expectation is that you will try to make contact with all of the patients. Should there be any patients whom you have not been able to contact, you are obliged to undertake some other action in the spirit of patient-centred care. For example, you should ensure that someone greets and apologises to the patients at reception, explaining that someone has tried to make contact with them, or you should inform the person who gave you the responsibility in the first place that you have not been able to make contact.

- If you say yes, whose responsibility is it to ensure that you clearly understand the expectation described above?
- What can you do or say to ensure you understand the task and its associated expectations before saying yes?

Authority

This refers to the level of 'power' that you have been given to make a decision in relation to a specific area of responsibility. It is a common area of misunderstanding and contention: you may either think that you have more authority than you have and be 'pulled back' or may not do as much as was expected of you because you did not realise that you had the authority to take a decision to implement a certain course of action. Authority is usually delegated to you, and so the level of authority that you have can be determined by someone else's philosophies and beliefs about what is reasonable for someone in your position to do, or by how accurate their knowledge and assessment of your abilities are.

Manthey and Miller (1994) propose four levels of authority and argue that it is helpful for all parties if the level of authority for a particular responsibility is clarified at the time that someone takes on the responsibility.

Table 3.3 Levels of authority

Level	Extent of authority
Level 1	Authority only to collect information that will then inform someone else in their decision-making process
Level 2	Authority to collect information and to make some recommendations that will then inform someone else in their decision-making process
Level 3	Authority to collect information, make some recommendations, then PAUSE to clarify purpose and understanding and then negotiate concerning the most appropriate recommendation to take forward and implement
Level 4	Authority to act and inform others after taking action

(adapted from Manthey and Miller, 1994)

The four levels are a helpful guide for clarifying the authority that you have for carrying out the obligations inherent within your responsibilities. The framework is also useful when you are in a position where you are delegating tasks and responsibilities to other people.

Level 4 can sometimes be misconstrued by some managers as 'Do as I would do'. In such instances, they have not really delegated level 4 authority, but level 3, as, in effect, they want you to pause and then implement the decision that they would have chosen as opposed to exercising your own judgement.

Accountability

Stereotypically, people think of being 'held' accountable, especially when something is perceived to have gone wrong and someone wants to know where the buck stops and who is responsible for this situation. This is a somewhat negative view and also infers that accountability is a retrospective action, something that you do to prove that you delegated appropriately or carried out the responsibility that you accepted in a reasonable manner. Instead, accountability should be a proactive and positive action. You should consider how you are going to demonstrate your accountability when you accept or delegate responsibility and authority; the principle would then be viewed in a more positive light.

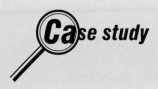
Case study

Accountability and assumptions

Jack, a newly qualified staff nurse asked Louise, a student nurse, who had just started her placement on a surgical ward, if she would check the temperature and blood pressure of all the post-operative patients at two-hourly intervals. Louise said yes and completed the task.

A little later when a patient was being reviewed, the doctor wanted to know why there was no record of post-operative observations. On Louise's last placement, an 'outpatient clinic,' patient observations were only recorded if they were outside of normal range, and she had applied the same principle on this ward, even though it was a very different environment providing very different care.

- What could Jack have done differently at the beginning that would have helped him to delegate in a more accountable manner?
- What could Louise have done differently that would have helped her to undertake the task in accordance with local ward procedures?
- What other factors might have contributed to the situation (e.g. time pressures, enthusiasm to be helpful, etc.)?

Reflective activity

Think of a time when you have been asked to do something and have agreed, without fully realising the implications.

- Whose responsibility was it to ensure that you understood what it was that you were being asked to do?
- With hindsight, what could you have done differently in order still to accept the responsibility but in a more robust manner?

Problem solving and decision making

Problem solving or decision making – decision making or problem solving? Is there a difference, does one come before the other or is it just a case of semantics? This chapter will take the pragmatic approach that similar processes, tools and techniques are applicable to both and that what differs is whether you see the situation as a problem to be solved or a situation that requires a decision to be taken. In the early stages of your health care career, you probably spend more time on identifying possible solutions to problems. Once you become a registered professional and gain more position power and authority, then you are likely to have to take more decisions regarding the best course of action to implement in order to address a particular situation or problem.

There are numerous tools and techniques to aid decision making, and these can be found both within the literature and via the Internet. We have chosen the following three for their ease of use, their combination of styles, their appropriateness for different situations and their ability to help you break through some of the brick walls that you might feel that you are facing with regard to some issues.

Upside-down technique

In essence, this technique is about doing the opposite and identifying all the ways that you know you would not use to resolve the problem.

- **Situation**. You have fallen out with another member of staff and now feel uncomfortable about working with them. You know you have to do something to address the situation, but what and how?
- **Technique**. Brainstorm all the words and ideas that come into your head that you know you should definitely **not** do with regard to this situation. This has two benefits. First, it is quite cathartic and allows you to let off steam by including all of those things you would like to say or do but know would do more harm than good. Secondly, having safely aired all the inappropriate options and clarified some of the potential 'grey' courses of action, it frees you up to identify constructive steps to move the situation forward. The process helps to sort out the clutter of what might or might not be a good idea and enables you to focus on what really needs to be done.

5 Whys model

This is an easy-to-use tool that allows for the complexity of what may at first appear to be a simple, single-problem event. Repeatedly asking 'Why did this happen?' can enable you to minimise the risk of only dealing with a symptom whilst increasing the likelihood of your dealing with the root cause and so creating a long-term solution. The goal is to get to the nub of the issue by gathering relevant information in order to be able to consider different courses of action before making a decision.

Consider the situation depicted in Table 3.4.

Table 3.4 The 5 Whys model in action

Situation	Drug dosage error occurs in the clinical room	
1. Why?	Staff Nurse A made an error in measuring the dosage	
2. Why?	The telephone in the clinic room was ringing	Receptionist had requested a phone be placed in the clinic room so that she could access a nurse urgently if she needed to
3. Why?	Because the receptionist wanted to pass a message on to the nurse	Receptionist had begun to phone for routine issues
4. Why?	Because a patient was insisting that she passed the message on *now*	Receptionist felt unable to deal with a patient who was being very insistent
5. Why?	Because the patient was parked in a restricted parking area	Very limited parking available for patients
Possible action	Remove telephone from clinic room Install a security alarm for emergencies	Training for receptionist on customer care strategies, basic de-escalation techniques Review of parking options

(adapted from Iles and Sutherland, 2001)

If you had stopped at the first 'why', the course of action might have included a disciplinary procedure for the drug error, attending a drug administration awareness session or a formal re-assessment of competence. However, as you work through each of the 'whys', it becomes evident that extra training for the staff nurse might have made no difference to the risk of the situation reoccurring. In this instance, once you have worked through the five whys, it becomes less and less likely that your interventions would focus solely on the staff nurse and more likely that you would instigate one or more of the possible action steps.

Reflective activity

Think of a situation that has occurred where, on the face of it, it was clear what had happened, who had made the mistake or how the mistake had occurred. Now apply the 5 Whys strategy to the situation and see if the process offers you any new insights or any new possible courses of action.

The Breakthrough Triangle

Similar to the upside-down technique, the Breakthrough Triangle involves breaking out of conventional ways of looking at a problem and coming up with possible ways of dealing with it from a position of having, mentally, already succeeded.

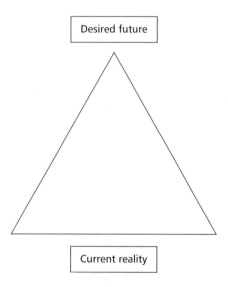

The Breakthrough Triangle

At the bottom of the triangle, you write a brief one-line descriptor of the current reality, such as 'I have six weeks to complete a 12,000-word thesis'.

At the top of the triangle, you write a brief and very specific one-line descriptor of the desired future, with a specific date for when it will be achieved: '1 November 2008 – I have completed my thesis to a high standard and submitted it on time'.

You then go mentally to that future date and say, 'I am there and I have done it. What did I do that enabled me to achieve my desired future?'

It is important to stay in the 'present' and, using the past tense, brainstorm 'What did I do?', writing the answers anywhere in or around the triangle. Keep asking yourself 'What else did I do?' until you feel that you have exhausted the brainstorm and then, looking at the points that you have written down, begin to prioritise them into what you think you did first, second, third, etc., in order to reach this point of success.

The result should be an action plan of what needs to be done in the order required to complete your thesis in six weeks' time. The outcome might not be revolutionary, but it should provide clarity and help to unblock some of the killer 'yes, but . . .' phrases that often arise when you are working from the present to the future. Everyone is usually very aware of what the difficulties are – the 'yes, buts . . .' that have to be

O━━┓ Keywords

Problem focused

Adopting a problem focus means that you keep narrowing down to get to the bottom of the situation (the 5 Whys strategy)

Solution focused

A solution focus is a more generative approach underpinned by the belief that there is probably a range of potentially useful options; it is just a case of identifying them and deciding which to do first (the Breakthrough Triangle strategy)

overcome – and very often we get slowed down or inhibited by them. By moving to a point in the future and saying, 'Well, we must have dealt with them, because we have reached our goal. Let's look at what it was we *must* have done that enabled us to overcome those potential blockages', you move from being **problem focused** to being **solution focused**.

Solution-focused techniques work best for issues that are within your influence or that you are part of and can contribute to the actions that need to be taken.

People often become so expert at identifying the problems that they find it difficult to step back and see potential solutions. The challenge is to avoid getting stuck in a rut of making decisions around perceived problems and to ensure that you also make decisions regarding the possibilities afforded by the future, which you may or may not yet know about. Von Oeck (1992) describes a leading business school that conducted a study which showed that its graduates did well at first, but, in 10 years, they were overtaken by a more streetwise, pragmatic group. The reason was that the first set of graduates had been taught how to solve problems, not how to recognise opportunities.

Reflective activity

What is your preferred approach to situations? Do you like to take a clear and logical approach and get to the bottom of a 'situation' or do you prefer to look at what 'could be' and whether there are any opportunities that could be explored?

You will no doubt be able to think of someone who, you feel, is always either 'problem focused' or 'opportunity focused', which restricts their ability to work effectively through some situations and often alienates some people around them owing to the 'single-mindedness' of their approach. Ideally, you need to be able to flex between the approaches so that you can adapt to the needs of the situation. (For more on solution-focused problem solving see Chapter 5, pp. 121–122.)

Prioritising your workload

Covey (1989) talks about the crux of effective management being the ability to 'put first things first': in other words, knowing how to prioritise the demands that are placed on you and being able to manage your time effectively so that you focus your energies on doing things that are important, which very often are not the things that are presented to you as being urgent.

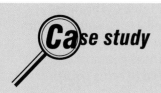

Important versus urgent

George had a real passion for patient-centred service development. He felt strongly that the patient's voice should have a stronger influence in the development of health care services. He had agreed with the senior nurse that he could have three hours the next Monday to go to the library and draft out some of his ideas in a format that could be presented to the clinical team. When Monday morning arrived, the service manager called the senior nurse to an urgent meeting. George was then told that he could not after all go to the library as the senior nurse could no longer 'cover' his workload.

- What issues does this situation highlight?
- Was it appropriate that George's time in the library was cancelled?
- How could George have dealt with the situation?
- How could the senior nurse have dealt differently with the situation?

In this instance, the work that George wanted to do was recognised by everyone as being important and in line with the strategic direction of the service. However, it was set aside for something 'urgent' that arose at short notice. This is a common challenge of effective time management. If we followed Steven Covey's (1989) mantra of 'first things first', then George's time would have been protected as what he was intending to do was recognised as being important. However, it was eclipsed by something else that was perceived as being urgent.

Some people are perceived as being very good in a crisis and, indeed, they appear to thrive on fire-fighting. There is always something happening around them. However, often they forget to pay attention to the things that are important but not yet a crisis and therefore neglect being proactive in the 'important:not urgent' section of the table and investing in service development and crisis avoidance. The consequence for them and staff can be 'burn-out' and reduced quality of patient care.

The more time that you can spend in 'important:not urgent', the more effectively you will use not just your time, but the time of others. By focusing your energies thus, you will not only get a higher return for your efforts, but for those around you as well. This section of the table is related less to problems and has more to do with possibilities and opportunities and what could be, which is a characteristic that Peter Drucker (2003) associates with effective managers. It is also a rewarding section to spend time in: somewhere you can refuel your passion for health care and the work that you do by investing time and effort into both the present and the future.

Table 3.5 Urgent vs. non-urgent issues

	Urgent	Not urgent
Important	Arise at short notice Crises Imminent deadlines Sometimes clinical-, often managerial-related Often could have been avoided with some forethought *Strategies* Delegate to the most appropriate person (which might be you) On completion, reflect on whether the crisis could have been avoided or minimised Reflect on what will not get done as a result of time spent in this section	Generally patient focused Ensuring important things become routine, e.g. good record keeping, standards of care Often practice or service development initiatives About being proactive About prevention of future crises Relationship-building initiatives – in team, with wider partners Innovative thinking and idea development *Strategies* Be clear about the importance of the activity and 'sell' that importance to others Plan time for priority activities in this section Time spent here is usually rewarding and helps to deliver on your fundamental values re. health care
Not important	Often arise at short notice Often described as urgent by someone in a more senior position Are often in response to someone else's agenda Interruptions – phone calls, emails, unplanned meetings Often visible and loud *Strategies* Clarify level of urgency Press the PAUSE button Does it have to be you who responds? Have a plan for the day; does the urgency of this issue override your plan for the day?	Trivial distractions – can be emails, phone calls, unplanned meetings Unproductive routine meetings Things you like doing, but are not really a good use of your time *Strategies* Look at emails once a day only Review the meetings that you attend. What is the cost–benefit of attending them? Review whether you should be delegating some of these activities Reflect on why you are spending time on things that are not important or urgent. Are you stressed, burnt out?

Reflective activity

Reflect on what you have done during the last week.

- In which of the four sections in Table 3.5 do you think you have spent most of your time and why?
- Could you have spent more time in the 'important:not urgent' section? If yes, what would you have to have done differently?
- Does your response to the previous question focus on what you could have done differently or has it drifted into 'If only they had . . .'-type statements?

Effective time management begins with you as an individual. If you want someone else to do something differently, then you need to identify what you could do that might result in the other person choosing to change their behaviour.

When are you at your most effective?

It is useful to ask yourself the questions listed in the following activity in order to understand your natural preferences and approaches.

Reflective activity

Take time to think about the following:

- What sorts of tasks do you work best at alone?
- At what stage in a task are you more effective when you:
  - work alone?
  - work with other people (e.g. when generating ideas, planning what needs to be done, implementing an action plan, following through to ensure everything has been seen to)?
- Are you a lark or an owl? – If you are a morning person and have a piece of work that requires a lot of concentration, then schedule it for a morning. If, however, you are an owl, and become more productive as the day goes by, then plan the piece of work for the afternoon.

Prioritisation

The matrix in Table 3.5 is a good framework for deciding on how to prioritise your time. In addition, several other strategies are recommended within the management literature.

One is to divide all demands on time into three categories:

- Don't do.
- Do later.
- Do now.

The challenge of this strategy is to build in a substantial amount of activity from the 'important:not urgent' section into the 'Do now' category.

In order to help you decide into which of the above categories an issue falls, Marquis and Huston (2000, p. 88) reiterate three key steps of time management, which are widely reflective of the core literature, namely:

1. Allow time for planning and establishing priorities.
2. Wherever possible, complete the highest-priority task first and endeavour to finish one task before beginning another.
3. Revisit your priorities based on the remaining tasks and on any new information that may have been received.

This last step is crucial in ensuring that you remain on track with regard to the direction in which you should be heading. If you have ever found yourself apparently out of step with others, it could be that you have forgotten to revisit the priorities and have not appreciated that a situation has changed and that, consequently, so have the priorities.

A priority change is often easier to determine when a clinical emergency arises: in Accident and Emergency (A&E), most people would recognise that an unconscious patient from a road traffic accident would take priority over a 15-year-old girl with a broken leg. However, managerial-type priorities, whether related to personal management or to team management are not always as clear to the less-experienced professional and, as a result, individuals are not always as flexible or responsive to changing situations.

Resource management

Resource management is about more than direct allocation or authorisation of money. We all have an individual responsibility to manage resources effectively and to appreciate the relationship between activity and resources. Resources can be actual money; however, time, equipment and running costs are also included, and each of us needs to seek to minimise any waste whilst maximising the utility or benefit that can be gained from what we are doing. In relation to your personal behaviours, resource management starts when you first become a student professional, and then continues to expand, when you become a first-line manager, to include the appropriate and judicious use of human, financial and other resources (Sullivan and Decker, 1997, p. 78).

Ask anyone about 'management' and their effective use of resources and you will generally elicit lots of stories about how wasteful they are and how much money could be saved if only we did things like this as opposed to that. Then ask them, 'So what have you done about it?' You generally get a long list of 'if only's' and 'I've tried, but . . .' or 'I'm only a student or a junior member of staff. No one will listen to me.'

Reflective activity

Spend five minutes reflecting on occasions during the last year when, you believe, time, money or other resources have been wasted.

Are you already saying to yourself, 'Yes, but I can't do anything about that because . . . I don't have the authority or the credibility or the boss doesn't like me' or you may have some other 'killer phrases' of your own to justify why you haven't done something about it.

A few key questions come to mind:
- How many times have you tried?
- Do you think that you have tried hard enough?
- How many different ways have you tried to raise the issue and get it addressed?
- What are the consequences of not getting it addressed, now, next month, next year?
- Do you have the necessary authority to address the issue?

Circle of Concern: Circle of Influence model

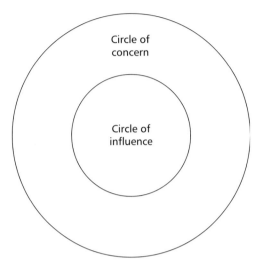

The Circle of Concern:
Circle of Influence model

Stephen Covey (1989) developed this model to demonstrate how you can either use your time and energy effectively to be proactive and focus your energies on what you can influence or you can get side-tracked by reacting to situations that you are concerned and frustrated about but very often cannot directly change. The latter is disheartening whilst the former, working in your 'circle of influence', is motivating because you are able to act and do something about the issue that is bothering you.

The challenge is to grow your circle of influence so that you increase the number of issues on which you can have a direct, positive impact.

To be effective, you need not only to recognise what lies within your circle of influence but equally importantly what lies within your circle of concern. You can then make a considered judgement as to how much energy to expend on something that you cannot directly influence. Alternatively, if it is sufficiently important, you can decide on what aspect of the issue you can bring into your circle of influence and do something about.

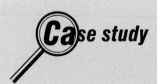

Achieving influence

Jack, a newly qualified nurse was convinced that a review of the current shift pattern on his ward could both save money and improve patient care by having fewer staff on at periods of low demand and higher staff numbers at times of higher patient demand. He had mentioned his idea a few times, but no one seemed very keen and there were always reasons as to why the shift pattern should stay as it was. Jack decided that he needed to convince a 'champion' who had a bigger circle of influence than he did. He mocked up three months' worth of staff rotas, using the proposed new shift system and, based on the demands of the previous three months, worked out the potential cost savings and then approached Gareth, the deputy charge nurse. Gareth was in charge of staff development and struggling to find the finances for the training and development needs of the ward. Jack's proposal did not have any obvious flaws and seemed like a possible solution to the training and development shortfall. Gareth tabled it for the next staff meeting when he showed how, if successful, the money saved would pay for a number of training courses that staff had requested; it might also offer more flexible working hours, as well as potentially improving patient care. It was agreed that there would be a three-month pilot of the new shift pattern, with a review one month in.

- How did Jack increase his circle of influence in order to get his proposal heard?

In the case study described above, Jack engaged someone with more position power and greater knowledge of the 'bigger picture'. As the deputy charge nurse in charge of staff development, Gareth knew that some members of staff were looking for increased flexibility in working hours, which Jack's proposal could potentially offer. Jack had seen that his proposal could be a possible solution to Gareth's problem and that this was likely to increase Gareth's motivation to listen to Jack's suggestion and give it a try. In turn, Gareth was able to present the proposal to the staff as a way of increasing the potential for individual staff members to access the training courses that they had requested, so motivating them sufficiently to override any feelings they might have that there was nothing wrong with the existing system.

Over to you

Revisit one of the issues you identified in the reflective activity on page 71 that needed addressing in relation to resource management. Using the Circle of Concern:Circle of Influence model, identify what is within your circle of influence and what you could do in order to increase that circle of influence and so increase the likelihood of your being able to make or instigate a change that would address the issue that you have identified.

Now for each possibility that you have identified, identify three practical steps that you could take that would be within your circle of influence.

Risk management

Risk refers to potential dangers, threats or perils and reducing their probability. McSherry and Pearce (2002, p. 36) advocate that, in the complex area of health care, risk should be viewed 'holistically, taking account of clinical, environmental and operational aspects of the service'.

The organisation in which you work is likely to have at least a Risk Manager and very probably a Risk Management department, so what is your role in risk management?

Over to you

Take 10 minutes and identify at least 5 points under each of the 3 broad categories of clinical, environmental and operational risk management (described below) where *you* have a responsibility for minimising potential threats.

Clinical risk management includes:

- ensuring that you are competent to take on a clinical procedure
- asking for advice and support when required in relation to clinical care
- initiating relevant procedures if you have a concern regarding another person's professional competence to practise safely.

Environmental risk management includes:

- contributing to maintaining an environment that is clean and safe (i.e. free from hazards) by, for example, moving a trailing wire as opposed to stepping over it
- reporting faulty equipment
- complying with COSHH requirements.

Operational risk management includes:

- implementing relevant policies and procedures – e.g. sickness, critical incident reports
- highlighting/reporting concerns in relation to safe staffing levels and suggesting possible solutions.

Awareness and training are important aspects of effectively contributing to risk management. One person will see a cracked plug and may wonder, 'How did that happen?' Someone else will recognise it as a potential hazard and either remove the plug or report the issue for immediate attention. The Department of Health (2000) document *An Organisation with a Memory* provides an excellent overview of the importance of everyone's contributing actively to the management of risk.

Quality improvement

What is quality management? What is actually meant by the term and how can it become something useful that you can engage with and not just another example of management-speak?

Moullin (2002) describes quality as being the way in which you (as an individual or part of an organisation) meet the requirements and expectations of service users and other stakeholders (public, staff, social services and other related organisations that service users come from and go to) whilst ensuring that costs are kept to a minimum. This implies an integrated approach to quality management that involves all parties and not just health care professionals and managers or someone who has 'quality' in their job title.

The importance of quality

- It is important for patients and service users
- It is important for staff
- It is important for resources. It can help to reduce costs and so provide an opportunity for an even better service in the resources available

Caruthers and Holland, cited in Moullin (2002), suggest that good quality may not always save money but poor quality always costs and usually wastes money and very often damages health.

One way of making the issue of 'quality' real for you as a practitioner is to examine the concept through 'dimensions of quality'. Maxwell's (1984) model, sometimes known as the 'A's and E's of quality' provides a useful six-point framework from which you can begin to determine the quality of the service that you are providing, either as an individual or as part of a team or a department. The six dimensions are:

- accessibility of the service by all who need it
- acceptability of the service to society, its users and stakeholders
- appropriateness or relevance of the service to the community
- effectiveness of the service for individuals
- equity and fairness of the service
- efficiency and economy of the service.

These dimensions are well established within health care and are embedded in *The NHS Performance Assessment Framework* (NHS Executive, 1999), which is a document that was intended to provide a coherent description of what it is that health services aim to offer service users and stakeholders.

Very often, professionals focus on the 'clinical' aspects of an acceptable service and forget about 'customer service' aspects of acceptability that are important to the service user.

Clinical Caseload . . .

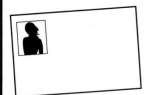

An outpatient renal dialysis service undertook a quality improvement audit and discovered that service users were irritated by the lack of available coat-hangers, which meant that they had to drape their clothes over the chair or fold them up and place them on the floor. Their comment: 'If I went to the hairdressers, they would always hang my coat up.' This was a quality improvement measure that was easy to implement and demonstrates that the quality improvement that service users ask for is often not related to major service reconfiguration or to spending lots of money but to basic customer care and being treated with respect and dignity as a person.

- What might be the value of sitting down and asking service users about their experience as opposed to giving them a questionnaire?
- What one thing could you do differently or better that would improve the quality of the experience for the service users with whom you interact?

A very useful strategy is to ask service users, carers and other stakeholders 'appreciative' questions about their experience. 'What do you like about the service you have received?' 'What has been helpful?' 'If there were three things that we should ensure that we keep doing, what would you recommend?' These types of 'appreciative' questions allow you to understand 'what is working' and 'what is important to service users'. Many of the areas highlighted are entirely predictable and include issues such as 'being made to feel welcome', 'feeling understood' and 'feeling safe', and 'understanding what was happening and likely to be happening in the near future'. In turn, these relate to such behaviours as clear and timely communication, both with the service users and their families and between professionals, and being spoken to and treated in a warm and respectful manner.

Appreciative inquiry involves moving away from noticing what is wrong or not working to noticing what is good and working well. It is founded on the principle that you get more of what you pay attention to. The approach creates a positive and uplifting environment that breeds in individuals and teams the confidence that they need to continue to improve their performance.

Appreciative questions create a very different dynamic from asking, 'What have you not been happy with or liked?' Also, this approach often makes it much easier for patients to be honest with us, whereas it is well documented that people tend to be unwilling to 'criticise' the service whilst they are still receiving it for fear of being 'penalised' in some way. Inviting people to provide appreciative feedback often lays the path for them to then feel able to say such things as 'You know what would have made it better, would have been if I could have seen the same physiotherapist each time' or '. . . if the health visitor could have visited at a time when my husband was at home'.

Keywords

Appreciative inquiry
Focuses on what it is that people or teams do well and explores how, if they did more of that or applied those skills elsewhere, they could be even better

Conclusion

As with leadership, there is no one right way to be a manager. However, you can develop good 'habits' underpinned by strong knowledge and skills, and the ideal time to start managing is before you become an 'identified' manager with specific management responsibilities.

This chapter has taken you through some core components of being an effective manager, with the emphasis being on self-management, beginning with self-awareness about your beliefs and thoughts and how those in turn influence your behaviour either positively or negatively.

If you are to be an effective manager, you need to understand who you are and the philosophy that underpins your management style. However, often we find it difficult to maintain a level of congruency between what we believe and how we behave. This is either because we feel pushed or pulled about by others or the system or because we have not thought clearly enough about the sort of managers that we want to be.

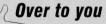

Over to you

- How does your underpinning philosophy show in your behaviour? Identify three examples.
- What sort of manager do you want to be? – Take a few minutes to write down some words that would begin to reflect this.
- Identify three specific skills that you would want to turn into good 'habits' in relation to you as a manager.

'People hear what we say, but they see what we do. And seeing is believing.' (anonymous)

RRRRRRapid recap

Check your progress so far by working through each of the following questions.

1. What is the difference between a 'reaction' and a 'response'?
2. Briefly define the concepts of 'care-taker' and 'rescuer'.
3. What type of time-management activities could be classed as 'important:not urgent'?
4. What is the value of working within your circle of influence as opposed to your circle of concern?
5. What are the six points of Maxwell's A's and E's quality framework?

If you have difficulty with more than one of the questions, read through the section again to refresh your understanding before moving on.

References

Adams, M. (2004) *Change Your Questions, Change Your Life: 7 Powerful Tools for Life and Work*. Berret-Koehler Publishers Inc., San Fransisco.

Blanchard, K., Oncken, W. and Burrows, H. (1994) *The One Minute Manager Meets The Monkey*. Harper Collins, London.

Covey, S. (1989) *The Seven Habits of Highly Effective People*. Simon & Schuster, Sydney.

Department of Health (2000) *An Organisation with A Memory*. The Stationery Office, London.

Harvey, E. and Lucia, A. (1995) *144 Ways to Walk the Talk*. Performance Publishing Company, Texas.

Iles, V. and Sutherland, K. (2001) *Managing Change in the NHS: Organisational Change a Review for Healthcare Managers, Professionals and Researchers*. NCCSDO, London School of Hygiene and Tropical Medicine, London.

Judge, T. and Watanabe, S. (1993) Another Look at the Job Satisfaction–Life Satisfaction Relationship. *Journal of Applied Psychology*. **78**(66): 939–948.

Manthey, M. and Miller, D. (1994) *Leading an Empowered Organisation Programme Manual*. Creative Healthcare Management, Minneapolis.

Marquis, B. and Huston, C. (2000) *Leadership Roles and Management Functions in Nursing – Theory and Application*. Lippincott Williams and Wilkins, Philadelphia.

Marriner-Tomey, A. (1996) *Guide to Nursing Management and Leadership*, 5th edn. Mosby, New York.

Maxwell, R. (1984) Quality Assessment in Health. *British Medical Journal*, **288** (12 May): 1470–1472.

McSherry, R. and Pearce, R. (2002) *Clinical Governance: A Guide to Implementation for Healthcare Professionals*. Blackwell Science, Oxford.

Moullin, M. (2002) *Delivering Excellence in Health & Social Care*. Open University Press, Buckingham.

NHS Executive (1999) *The NHS Performance Assessment Framework*. Department of Health, The Stationery Office, London.

Sullivan, E.J., and Decker, P.J. (1997) *Effective Management in Nursing*, 4th edn. Addison Wesley, Harlow.

Van Oech, R. (1992) *A Whack on The Side of The Head – How You Can Be More Creative*. Creative Think, California.

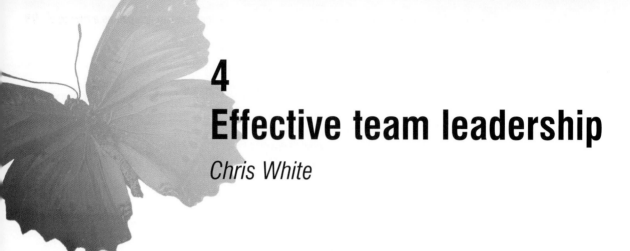

4
Effective team leadership

Chris White

Learning outcomes

By the end of this chapter you should be able to:

★ Define the purpose of teams

★ Outline the characteristics of a team

★ Define different types of teams

★ Recognise team learning

★ Identify leadership as everybody's business

★ Understand reactions and responses

★ Discuss the implications of change to organisational structures

★ Explain team members' behaviour in terms of effective and non-effective leadership

★ Use effective behaviours in less-than-perfect situations

★ Understand the causes of poor performance in teams.

Overview of the theory

> The activity of a group of people working co-operatively to achieve shared goals via differentiation of roles and using elaborate systems of communication is basic to our species. The current enthusiasm for teamworking in health care reflects a deeper, perhaps unconscious, recognition that this way of working offers the promise of greater progress than can be achieved through individual endeavour or through mechanistic approaches to work.
>
> Borrill et al. (2002, p. 230)

Leadership is a set of behaviours that can be learnt equally by people in formal management positions and by people who do not think of themselves as leaders. Most of us have leadership challenges in our day-to-day lives in individual and small-group interactions; we use the skills of a salesperson, the credibility of a trusted friend, and occasionally the courage of a freedom fighter (Bergmann et al., 1999, pp. 1–2). This can apply equally when working with service-users and their carers or when working as part of a team to deliver the service.

What is a team?

All human interaction is about cooperating with other people. The way we express our individuality and what we have in common is through groups such as families, and social and work organisations (West and Markiewicz, 2004, p. 2).

Leading a team and ensuring that the team maximises its shared knowledge, experience and skill is very different from traditional supervision (West and Markiewicz, 2004, p. 8). Everyone can do this, not just the person with the title 'leader'.

Characteristics of a team

- Team members share objectives.
- They have the necessary authority, autonomy and resources to achieve these objectives.

- They have to work closely and interdependently to achieve these objectives.
- They have well-defined and unique roles.
- They are recognised as a team.
- A team includes no fewer than 3 and no more than 15 members (West and Markiewicz, 2004, p. 11).

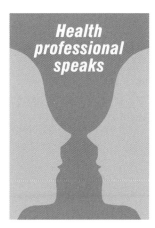

Health professional speaks

Team Leader NHS

In my area of work in rehabilitation, in the hospital, there is one team in which staff are from the same discipline but work independently in a wide variety of specialist areas. They are known as a team because they are all managed by one person.

In contrast, in the community, a team of multi-professionals share the same caseload: although they are all line-managed by their own professions, their work is interdependent and their objectives are shared.

Team leadership is:

- Creating agreement around shared objectives and strategies to achieve them
- Helping people appreciate each other and helping them to learn how to confront and resolve differences constructively
- Helping people to coordinate activities, continuously improve, develop their capabilities, encourage flexibility, encourage an objective analysis of processes, and foster collective learning about better ways to work together
- Representing the interests of the group or organisation, protecting its reputation, helping to establish trust with external stakeholders
- Helping to resolve conflicts between internal and external partners
- Creating a unique group identity

(adapted from Borrill *et al.*, 2002, pp. 221–222)

Over to you

Read the material in the box above describing team leadership and, for each of the characteristics listed, identify ways that you can be an effective 'follower'. Now read the material again, identifying how you can lead in that area in relation to your patients as stakeholders and partners, your colleagues in a workplace, or your family and friends.

What do you mean by 'team'?

Sometimes, the words 'group' and 'team' are used interchangeably. 'Team' may refer to workers with specific functions or autonomous shop-floor working arrangements. Sometimes, it is used to mean a collection of people as they should be, or would prefer to be, rather than what they actually are (Buchanan and Huczynski, 2004, p. 307).

Definitions of teams

Defining the type of team you are in is not nearly as important as the members contributing to common objectives; in reality, it can be surprising that neither of these issues is explored and understood in teams. Being a team may be nothing more significant than a convenient label. Terminology can be misleading as the same term may mean different things.

Here are some explanations based on dictionary definitions of commonly used terms:

- **multi-disciplinary**: many or much; many disciplines together; often used as a term to describe a meeting, such as a case conference, where parallel professions or agencies meet, usually at a particular point in time in the patient journey
- **intra-disciplinary**: within, on the inside; suggests comprising different disciplines with set boundaries; perhaps intended to mean fewer disciplines or more closely related ones – in terms of a specific condition – than in a multi-disciplinary team
- **inter-disciplinary**: between, among, mutually, reciprocally; suggests that roles have been defined by core skills of each discipline and that there is blurring of professional boundaries in areas of commonality
- **network teams/pathway**: a chain of interconnected persons, operations, etc.; suggests that this is over time, through the patient journey and that this is coordinated and managed in terms of norms and variances
- **interagency teams**: simply suggests that team members are employed by different agencies. This may or may not be a problem, depending on the amount of time that the members spend together and the consequent strength of their relationships and allegiances.

Definitions of team performance

- **Working group**: members interact primarily to share information and views, coordinate practices, etc. There is little shared responsibility – the emphasis is on individual responsibility, and there is no significant need or opportunity requiring it to become a team

- **Pseudo-team**: not really focused on communal responsibility and coordination and is not trying to achieve it. Less impact than working groups because interactions detract from members' individual performance without delivering any joint benefits

- **Potential team**: trying to improve performance impact, but lacks clarity about shared goals and individual accountability to the team and working practices

- **Real team**: a small group of people with complementary skills, who are equally committed to a common purpose, goal and working approach, for which they hold themselves mutually accountable

- **High-performance team**: a group that meets all the conditions of real teams and has members who are deeply committed to each other's personal growth and success (Katzenback and Smith, 1993, p. 91)

- **Virtual teams**: 'virtual' implies that the common workplace is via technology, meaning that team members may be in the same (co-located) or different (distributed) locations so that their communication and information sharing may be synchronous (at the same time) or asynchronous (in different time zones). The combination of advances in communication and increasing globalisation and competition means that individuals anywhere in the world can interact on the move and share information (Buchanan and Huczynski, 2004, p. 309)

- **Self-directed teams**: teams that share the leading rather than having one single leader; the person best suited to the task takes the lead. The evaluation of performance and achievement of goals is by mutual accountability. In discussion about the training of marines, Katzenbach and Santamaria describe how the groups are highly cohesive and are able to learn when to use real team and single-leader team to best advantage (Buchanan and Huczynski, 2004, p. 308)

Reflective activity

Think about all of the teams with which you are involved within work/study and at home.

- What is the purpose of these teams? What do they exist to do?
- Is there agreement on the purpose from all the members?

Can a team learn?

Because teams are the basic unit in organisations, where 'the rubber hits the road', organisations are unable to learn if teams do not (Senge, 1990 p. 10).

Team learning is about building relationships that are open to lifelong learning, being prepared to give and take, and opening up our deepest thoughts and beliefs to challenge – suspending judgement and learning to put defensiveness to one side. This is a discipline that requires practice to master. We will never arrive at the end of it because the more we learn, the more we realise what we do not know (Senge, 1990, p. 10).

By being prepared to think new thoughts, we can identify problems and potential solutions that none of us could have thought of alone.

Everyone is a leader

Opportunities for leadership for everyone can be ambiguous, poorly defined and not without risk. To be successful, people often have to go outside what they are used to in terms of location and comfort zones. Policies and procedures may need to be questioned and people higher up in the organisation asked to provide more information, clarify issues, and make difficult decisions (Bergmann *et al.*, 1999, p. 3).

There are many reasons why people take such challenging opportunities: because they want to make their own and others' jobs easier, feel a strong sense of ownership, seek recognition or advancement or want to make an impact. Sometimes, it is because of a heartfelt conviction that it is simply the right thing to do: and sometimes it is because of a complex interplay of unexamined reasons, because you know that, if you do not, there is no one who will (Bergmann et al, 1999, p. 4).

Flattening of hierarchical organisational structures also creates leadership opportunities. There are fewer managers and supervisors than there used to be, and those who are left have taken on extra responsibilities and may be compromised in their leadership duties (Bergmann *et al.*, 1999, p. 7).

Evidence base

Read Peters, T. and Waterman, R.H. (eds) (2004) *In Search of Excellence*. Profile Books, London.

It was not intended that Peters and Waterman's research would become a book, but it has turned out to be a classic text. Peters has said that the essential message became:

- people
- customers
- action.

It was probably the beginning of the realisation that 'soft' factors are highly important in business; this theme is still very current in the age of consumerism and customer choice.

The eight themes form the titles of the chapters:

- a bias for action – active decision making – 'getting on with it'
- close to the customer – learning from the people served by the business
- autonomy and entrepreneurship – fostering innovation and nurturing 'champions'
- productivity through people – treating rank and file employees as a source of quality
- hands-on, value-driven – management philosophy that guides everyday practice – management showing its commitment
- stick to the knitting – stay with the business that you know
- simple form, lean staff – some of the best companies have minimal HQ staff
- simultaneous loose-tight properties – autonomy in shop-floor activities plus centralised values.

Evidence base

Read Covey, S. (1992) *Principle-centred Leadership*. Simon and Schuster, London.

Principle-centred Leadership follows on from *The Seven Habits of Highly Effective People* (Covey, 1989) and focuses on the conflicts and dilemmas that do not respond to quick fixes. Covey applies 'the law of the farm': prepare the ground; plant the seed; cultivate; weed; water it; nurture growth and development to full maturity. These natural laws and principles operate whether we recognise them or not and we should look to centre ourselves around them if we want to be effective.

On page 107 of *Principle-centred Leadership*, Covey lists 10 'power tools' that raise honour, respect and regard from others:

- persuasion – sharing reasons and rational, genuine respect for the ideas and perspective of others; committing to continue to communicate until mutually beneficial and satisfying outcomes are reached

- patience – with processes and people; keep a long-term perspective and stay committed to goals in the face of short-term obstacles and resistance
- gentleness – with the feelings and vulnerabilities of others
- teachableness – remember that you do not have all the answers and insights; value different viewpoints, judgements and experiences
- acceptance – give the benefit of the doubt; withhold judgement and remember that everybody's self-worth is important
- kindness – remember to nurture relationships: being sensitive and caring: little things are the big things
- openness – get accurate information and perspectives of others regardless of what they own, control or do; consider their intentions, desires, values and goals – do not only focus on their behaviours
- compassionate confrontation – in the context of genuine care, concern and warmth, acknowledge mistakes and errors so that it is a safe environment in which to take risks
- consistency – stick to your values and character; do not manipulate when you do not get your way or are faced with a crisis
- integrity – desire the good of others; match your words and feelings with thoughts and actions, without malice, desire to deceive, take advantage, manipulate or control.

Building legitimate power by the person you are influences others without force and brings peace of mind from knowing that you are becoming wiser and more effective.

Politics

Politics is about balancing what you want to achieve with what is going on in the team and the bigger picture. Reeves (1998, p. 152) describes it as the natural process of getting things done and the tendency that we all have to be influenced and directed by our values and needs or by external conditions such as cultural norms and other people's expectations.

Empowerment

'Power', like politics, is a concept with a poor image – mainly for the same reasons. Because it has connotations of domination and coercion, some people like to think that they do not have or use it. More acceptable neutral terms such as 'authority' or 'influence' may be used to describe the ability to get other people to do things. However, as well as control or command over other people, power can mean having liberty or permission to act; and this is the meaning of 'empowerment'.

As discussed in Chapter 2, there are different types of power: power that goes with your position – formal authority – and personal power that comes, for example, from your particular expertise or knowledge.

Related to power is your capacity to shape events. So use of power includes all the various means by which you get things done through other people, from coercing, through influencing to giving others freedom to exercise their own power (Reeves, 1998, pp. 206–207).

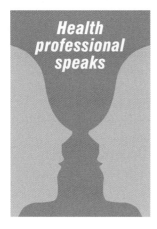

Health professional speaks

Health care assistant

When new staff start work in our team I take them under my wing and show them round, where to find things, how things are done around here, who to ask if you need something.

I have lots of experience and skills; sometimes that is appreciated and other times qualified staff don't want my opinion. We can both learn, and the patients will benefit even more if we can both add our different expertise together.

Reflective activity

Think of people who are influential without formal authority – for example, Ghandi, Mother Teresa, and Martin Luther King.

● What was it that made people listen to them?

● Can you identify if these are the same reasons why you have respect for others?

● How can you cultivate these qualities in your work?

Consensus

When people think of consensus, they often think of everyone changing their views to those of the most convincing person within the team. Sometimes, this is the case but, more often, the process of discussion and presenting different points of view leads to new avenues of thought and alternatives that no one person had discovered. So there are two purposes to discussion: to diverge, not seeking agreement but to understand better all the issues; and to focus down on a conclusion, having weighed alternative views (Senge, 1990, p. 247).

Johnson and Scholes (2002, p. 52) note that the environment is complex and rapidly changing so that it is unlikely, and probably not desirable, that everyone should agree. Although it is not always comfortable, a diversity of ideas and views encourages innovation because it challenges assumptions and encourages experimentation. New ideas are most likely to succeed where they are allowed and encouraged to compete with each other.

Consultation

It is a common problem in the cascade of information to teams that the purpose of the communication is unclear. If there is a belief that consensus is always the right thing then people may think that their opinions are being sought when, in fact, there is no option and the change must happen. Organisations do have to comply with policies and directives; sometimes, there is no choice, and compliance cannot be negotiated.

However, there may be choice in the way that change is implemented, and this may be decided by the team if members are able to be proactive rather than reactive to enforced change.

Another reason why consensus may not be sought is that it is very time consuming; if decisions have to be made quickly, it may be impossible to consult.

Proactive or reactive?

Oshry (1996, p. 103–110) describes how, in many systems, societies or organisations, people categorise themselves as dominant or dominated. This is not as simple as minorities being dominated, because majorities may also behave as if dominated, and minorities may behave as dominators, oppressing the dominated. If we perceive ourselves to be dominated, we have several options to use as coping strategies; Oshry (1996) calls this 'the dance of power' and identifies the following coping behaviours:

- adopt – try to behave like the dominators by imitating their culture
- embrace – accept it as our fate; choose it and get on with it
- separate – keep away from them and reject their ways; have our own culture
- rebel – try to destroy the dominant culture; discredit it; try to dominate 'them'
- drop out – withdraw from both cultures; drop out into alcohol, drugs, etc.
- crime – since the dominant culture is unfair, break 'their' laws, steal, cheat, lie, get what we can
- transform – embrace both cultures and customs, value both histories and spirituality.

Transformation is not easy, because the dominated culture is not perceived as an option by dominators – they think that their way is the only one and may be offended that others believe that there is a choice.

I am sure that you can think of many examples of these options in society in your own country, and they are certainly evident in the war-torn scenes that we see on the televised news from around the globe.

It may be harder to apply this concept in the workplace, but, if you become more aware, you will notice 'dominated' behaviours within teams that perpetuate old problems and behaviours. Transformation is a possibility here too, but there may be resistance from both sides.

Reflective activity

Do you think that people living in Berlin before the wall came down, or women not allowed to vote, would have thought that transformation was possible?

Essential team leadership behaviours

Having looked at some theoretical aspects of leadership, we will now look at essential team leadership behaviours, the behaviours needed by everyone for effective team outcomes.

Knowledge, skills and abilities

If a team is to achieve its goal, all team members need certain attributes (Borrill *et al.*, 2002, p. 219). The quality of the teamworking is directly related to the outcomes for patients (Borrill *et al.*, 2002).

Table 4.1 Knowledge, skills and abilities for teamworking

A Knowledge, skills and abilities for conflict resolution	Fostering useful conflict, while eliminating dysfunctional conflict. Using win–win strategies rather than win–lose strategies
B Knowledge, skills and abilities for collaborative problem solving	Having the right level of participation for any given problem; managing obstacles to team problem solving (e.g. domination by some team members)
C Knowledge, skills and abilities for communication	Using an open and supportive style of communication that maximises an open flow. Using active listening techniques. Paying attention to non-verbal messages
D Knowledge, skills and abilities for goal setting	Setting specific, challenging and attainable team goals. Monitoring, evaluating and providing feedback on performance
E Knowledge, skills and abilities for planning and task coordination	Coordinating and synchronising tasks, activities and information. Establishing fair and balanced roles and workloads among team members

(adapted from Stevens and Campion (1999) in Borrill (2002, p. 22))

Strategies for change

The CLIMB model describes the five leadership strategies that outstanding executives follow to ensure the success of an organisational change initiative:

Create a compelling future

Let the customer drive the organisation

Involve every mind

Manage work horizontally

Build personal credibility

(Bergmann *et al.*, 1999, p. 11).

This model of leadership is 'grassroots' because it is rooted in behaviours that can be performed by anyone, no matter what their position.

The leader in each of us

CLIMB strategies	Competencies
Create a compelling future	Creating and communicating a vision Managing changes required to make vision reality
Let the customer drive the organisation	Responding to customer identified needs
Involve every mind	Supporting individual and team efforts Sharing information Making decisions that solve problems
Manage work horizontally	Managing processes across functions Good use of technical skills Managing projects Managing time and resources
Build personal credibility	Taking initiative beyond the job requirements Taking responsibility for your own actions and the actions of your group Handling emotions in yourself and others Displaying professional ethics Showing compassion Making credible presentations

(adapted from Bergmann *et al.*, 1999, p. 15)

These behaviours define leadership competencies. They are not traits, such as tenacity or integrity, which are often thought of as characteristics of effective leaders. This distinction is important because it is possible to learn specific behaviours, like sharing information, but it is much more difficult to develop, or to describe how to develop openness or honesty, for example (Bergmann *et al.*, 1999, p. 14).

The CLIMB model defines leadership, not just for executives, but also for all employees. Using CLIMB, you can evaluate your leadership if you are an executive, front-line worker or anywhere in between. More importantly, it is possible to improve leadership by training in the competencies summarised by CLIMB. In other words, 'there is a leader in each of us' (Bergmann *et al.*, 1999, p. 16).

Practical ways to see vision

There is agreement in the literature that a vision is essential in leadership (Bergmann *et al.*, 1999; Peters and Waterman, 2004) but there is more to it than deciding a personal vision that may be different from others. Practical ways of defining vision are helpful because the idea of vision is sometimes discredited as not being practical or grounded in reality. Using the question 'What do you aspire to?' may be more acceptable. Possibilities include:

- **Story boarding.** Assembling random pictures from magazines and describing how each picture connects to what you are doing or aspiring to releases the power of the subconscious mind and enables creative thinking in order to move forward out of ruts.

- **A picture**. A garden, a pond or bench to sit on can be used as a metaphor for stopping to reflect. A plant or tree can represent growth: the fruit and the roots will all have significance for what you are doing in your team, and so on. Pictures have an inherent meaning for individuals, without the misunderstandings caused by particular words.

The benefits of visual representation of what your team sees as its purpose are:

- building cohesion
- identifying what you need to achieve
- checking out common values and aspirations
- a trademark
- building rapport.

> ### Over to you
>
> Further ideas for creativity and flexible thinking are available in many books and Internet resources, try a search!
>
> Here are a few to get you started:
> www.creativityatwork.com
> www.edwdebono.com
> www.directedcreativity.com.

How can we tell a good team?

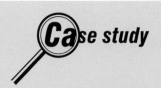

An example of a team's self-assessment

At a time of organisational change, a team used the Team Process Questionnaire – a simplified version of the Team Climate Inventory© (West and Markiewicz, 2004, p. 135) – to identify their strengths and areas for development in five essential behaviours for effective teamworking. This enabled them confidently to take their best practice in commitment to team objectives, support and participation forward into the new work environment and to develop constructive debate and innovation, enhancing job satisfaction and quality of service.

● Are all five of the essential behaviours: commitment to team objectives, support, participation, constructive debate and innovation present in your team?

● Can you identify objective examples that illustrate each of the five behaviours?

● How would your colleagues rate the team against the five behaviours?

● How can you raise awareness of areas that could be improved?

If, rather than being interviewed for what you bring to a team, you were able to interview the team you wanted to work with, what would your criteria be: environment and surroundings, team behaviours or just intuition?

It is very difficult to be objective, but, when applying for a job, it is good to look round before interview; this will give you more confidence, and you should formulate questions for the interviewers to check out your assumptions and to get a more objective feel of the team.

Formal ways of evaluating teams are available from many perspectives, as a baseline measure or as a way of evaluating changes by auditing an aspect of team function. Remember when judging a team by one measure that all human interactions are complex and interrelating.

Recognised questionnaires are available to evaluate, at team level specifically, team functioning and performance, autonomy, team climate and team process, innovation, satisfaction and reflexivity (see West and Markiewicz, 2004, pp. 120–152, for resources). Some of these are complex in analysis, allow comparison with norms and require payment to process; others are simple and free. The strength of your trust in the results should be tempered accordingly, but even simple questionnaires can give an indication.

Core Competency of Clinical Teams identifies and rates competency statements in terms of their importance and personal current performance (Allen and Pickering, 2002). Although this lacks the rigor of **360° evaluation**, it has been shown that poor performing areas have recognised problems, but the individuals who knew did not understand the implications or find alternatives (Senge, 1990, p. 17). We can suppose that it is not difficult to tell that there is a problem, although doing something about it is a different matter. However, recognition is always the first step to finding a solution.

🔑 Keywords

360° evaluation
Is a review taken from many perspectives, your own, other team members, service users, your boss

Core competencies of clinical teams

Competency statements

1. Patient and/or carer focus: establish and maintain effective relationships with patient and/or carers

    1a Establish and maintain effective two-way relationships with patients

    1b Enable patient and/or carers to make informed decisions

    1c Contribute to and support the decision-making process

2. Team focus: establish and maintain effective team delivery

    2a Understand the range of roles within service-delivery team and how their strengths and limitations can contribute to effective patient care

    2b Assume service team leadership in decision making

    2c Contribute to the development of an effective team ethos and vision

3. Interpersonal understanding and impact: identify and understand others' needs and concerns and modify own response to build credibility, mutual respect and trust

    3a Establish and maintain effective relationships with team members

    3b Maintain personal stability when under pressure

4   Quality assurance: contribute to the process of continuous improvement in patient and/or carers' care

    4a Commitment to improve own performance in order to improve the delivery of patient care

    4b Review team performance in order to improve the delivery of patient care

(adapted from Allen and Pickering, 2002)

These competencies show that the competency of teams is dependent on the behaviours of each member; everyone is responsible for their own contribution. As you can see, each statement is accompanied by performance indicators that spell out the behaviours that evidence competency.

Over to you

Look through the competencies and identify and write down your own areas for development. Seek out supervision or mentorship to discuss how you can set objectives to work on these areas. Is there someone in your team who could be asked to remind you of your commitment to change if they observe old behaviour?

My own initial experiences of leadership were using Practice Development Accreditation with the Centre for the Development of Healthcare Policy and Practice (for more information, visit the website at www.cdhpp.leeds.ac.uk) at the University of Leeds. Practice Development Accreditation uses 15 criteria formed into a multi-dimensional and interconnecting framework for assessing and developing practice. We used this approach to change from Care of the Elderly, establishing the speciality of Rehabilitation over a two-year period, and subsequently maintaining and continuing to develop practice with re-accreditation.

Reflective activity

- Can you identify a challenge that your team is facing that would benefit from a framework approach to guide development?
- Will the challenge lend itself to a single-dimension approach (such as quality improvement) or does it have many facets?

What to do in a less-than-perfect team

So what can you do if you are working in a less-than-perfect team? Maybe you feel like the only one who cares at the moment. If this is the case:

- Keep reminding yourself of the vision/purpose.
- Write down the reasons why you took the job/profession, renewing your passion.
- Seek to understand, check out assumptions.
- Seek out supervision or mentoring.
- Lead by example, for example model good time management and professional appearance.
- Reinforce all positives, possibilities, opportunities and potential.
- Do not reciprocate practices that you want to end.

Oshry (1996, p. 69) disputes that it 'takes two to tango': he says that we can, as individuals, learn a new dance; you may be dancing alone for a while, but you create the possibility of change by breaking the pattern. In the short term, this may feel messy and chaotic, but remember that change does feel uncomfortable and that you need to stick with it or the old routines will simply reinstate themselves.

Gently challenge constant negativity; silence is agreement – we promote what we permit (Halligan, 2003). This is one step more than only being responsible for your own behaviour: it is hard to deal with something that has been condoned; the longer you leave it, the harder it is to challenge. It may be the case that, because something has not been challenged, the people involved do not even recognise that it is happening, or that it is considered by others to be inappropriate.

Remember, health care environments are complex and many factors are involved. However, it takes one brave person, standing up for their principles, to begin the process of change.

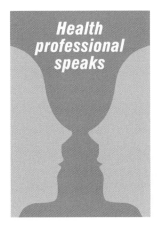

Health professional speaks

Nurse

It sounds really awful but I didn't even think how I would feel if it was me; we had just always done it that way. It wasn't until one of my patients asked if we could find a way of them being able to be independent with flushing the toilet that I realised how embarrassing it must be for them. I had always thought it was OK for me to do it for them because I'm a nurse.

Think of saying no as a beginning of something new, rather than focusing on the discomfort that the end of something brings. It can be conversation starting; Oshry (1996, p. 86) thinks of resistance as the sound of the familiar dance shaking.

Issues used to be passed up the chain of command, to be sorted out higher up. Now, with networking through our patient's journey, it is front-line staff who build relationships and sort out issues themselves (Allee, 2003, p. 16).

Research shows that there are common themes when things go wrong and are left to become really serious. The following box highlights these.

Common themes of inquiries

Organisational or geographical isolation – which inhibits the transfer of innovation and hinders peer review and constructive critical exchange

Inadequate leadership – lacking vision and unwilling to tackle known problems

System and process failure – in which organisational systems and processes are either not present at all or not working properly

Poor communication – both within National Health Service organisation and between it and patients or clients, which means that problems are not picked up

Disempowerment of staff and patients – which means that those who might have raised concerns were discouraged or prevented from doing so.

(Walshe and Higgins, 2002)

Everyone is responsible

I am sure that everyone can recognise some of these issues in their workplace. Frequently, there are longstanding issues that existing team members feel are impossible to tackle.

There is growing awareness of 'corporate citizenship': all of us have a responsibility. Accordingly, we have broken complex problems down into manageable chunks and, as a result, have lost the big picture so that we are unable to see the consequences of our actions (Senge, 1990, p. 3).

Reflective activity

Next time you are tempted to pretend that you did not notice something – telling yourself that it is nothing to do with you – remember that you are a global citizen. What are you condoning by doing nothing? What will the consequences of that be?

Where is the problem?

A different way of thinking – a new way to perceive our world and ourselves – is to see ourselves as connected to the whole, not separate from it. We no longer see the problem as 'out there', but begin to understand how our actions create the problems that we experience (Senge, 1990, p. 12).

It is our decision. However exciting and invigorating taking charge of your own destiny is, there are always some who remain committed to their old ways, whining, complaining, and more committed to blaming others and feeling victimised than to success (Oshry, 1996, p. 73). Trusting managers to sort issues out for us is a prelude to blaming them when things do not turn out as we wanted (Oshry, 1996, p. 75).

Do remember that change takes time and that there is an overlap period. You can expect to see contradictions, when the talk is about the new order of things but business appears as usual because the thinking is still of the old order (Allee, 2003, pp. 19 and 38).

As we begin to understand other people's worlds, we can see how our own actions have made it difficult for others to cooperate with us, and see how we might get what we need by helping each other instead of making things worse (Oshry, 1996, p. 23).

Working for partnership

Our inability to see ourselves and to see the actions we take as they really are leads us out of the possibilities of partnership and into opposition, antagonism and disappointment. It is up to us, from whatever side of each relationship we are in, to stop unproductive, and often destructive, familiar behaviours and transform them into ones that are more satisfying and constructive (Oshry, 1996, p. 51).

What often gets in the way of new possibilities is a feeling of 'self righteousness': we feel that the other person should make the first move because we think that they are wrong. To be constructive, put that aside and concentrate on what it is that needs to happen, looking for 'win–win' opportunities.

Structured reflection on team behaviours

On more than one occasion, I have heard stories about the expectations of customers or service users booking a flight. When you book an aeroplane journey, it is not usual to check the qualifications of the pilot; you take that for granted. You judge the quality of the journey purely on customer service: the food, the manner and appearance of the crew, their courtesy, and if they greet you and smile.

It is absolutely no different in health care. The human touches, going the extra mile to ensure that someone is comfortable, the tone of your voice, the time you take, giving your full attention: these are the things that improve customer satisfaction and make them want to choose to come back.

Sensing possibilities

We must stop looking for one answer and start sensing patterns, fostering dynamic relationships and exploring interdependencies (Allee, 2003, p. 15). Our lives are made up of a web of relationships (Oshry, 1996, p. 101). When we do not see the whole system, all we see are individual personalities. Our explanations and our solutions are personal (Oshry, 1996, p. 167).

It isn't simple

Unconsciously, we try to stretch our old perspective and ways of doing things to encompass new ideas (Allee, 2003, p. 38). This adds to the mess and lack of clarity. There may also be paradox – when two apparently opposing statements can both be true – our experience of something leads us to a view of it that may not be so in other circumstances (Allee, 2003, p. 95).

We do have a tendency to think that something is either this or that, when in fact it can be both this and that (Bate, 1995, p. 28). It is commonly thought that differences cannot be tolerated, when in fact there is new strength in teams that recognise that many divergences are creatively compatible and that partnerships can produce working that is much better than only doing one thing or the other (Oshry, 1996, p. 173).

We pressure ourselves by thinking that teams must all do the same thing all the time; thus differences that could coexist become enemies to one another. This is a destructive illusion (Oshry, 1996, p. 177).

Our old ways were not wrong, but just too small. They become the foundations of our new thinking; as we come across anomalies that current reasoning cannot explain, exploring serves as a gate to the next level of understanding, and questions are important to move us forward (Allee, 2003, p. 39). It is exploring others' perspectives that helps us to see where our explanation of something is incomplete; this is the power of asking others, whether within the team or from other areas, new members of staff and, especially, service users.

It is your choice

There are some interesting studies of health care environments. One, cited by Goleman *et al.* (2003, p. 21), took place in cardiac care units and found that, if the nurses' general mood was 'depressed', the death rate among patients was four times higher than on comparable units.

Borrill *et al.* (2002) studied some 400 health care teams and showed that the quality of teamwork directly and positively relates to the quality of patient care and innovation, and directly and negatively relates to mortality rates in hospitals: good teamwork saves lives.

There are many references cited to support the idea that the emotions that people experience are what holds them together in a team and causes commitment to organisations (Goleman *et al.*, 2003, p. 17).

I can certainly agree from personal experience that, when I feel valued and listened to, and when I perceive that the organisation is pursuing things that are important to me, I feel a great sense of pride and belonging. I believe that this is one of the important reasons for using supervision in the workplace: that we can speak about what is troubling us, what is important and get someone else's 'take' on the situation to increase our understanding. This is what builds teamwork in its broadest sense – being understood and being able to contribute.

Reflective activity

Think of a time when you have had a moan after a meeting. What questions could you have asked during the meeting to gain a better understanding of the reasons behind the situation? How could you use supervision to share your feelings and build coherence?

It is the relationships between people that make situations go excellently, well, or badly for the 'customer'. Your own experience will tell you this – when everyone gets on well and tries to help each other out, it is much smoother than when staff are distracted by bickering and 'that's not my job' attitudes.

We all have experience of friendships that we consider healthy: the characteristics are open and honest communication, trust, mutual respect, and reliable support.

Covey (1989) thinks of our interactions with each other as being like an emotional bank account:

> If I make deposits into an Emotional Bank Account with you through courtesy, kindness, honesty and keeping my commitments to you, I build up a reserve. Your trust toward me becomes higher, and I can call upon that trust many times if I need to. I can even make mistakes and that trust level, that emotional reserve, will compensate for it.
>
> Covey (1989, p. 188)

Teams make better decisions than individuals but not if the team lacks harmony and members are not cooperative with each other. Everyone in a group contributes to the emotional intelligence of a group; emotions are contagious, and it is useful to step back and look at what the group has adopted as its 'norm' or team culture. These are the unspoken ground rules, for instance contention and confrontation or a thin veneer of civility and interest or, in more effective teams, respect, listening, questioning, support and working through disagreements (Goleman *et al.*, 2003, pp. 223–226).

Here is a mandate for effective team behaviours.

Commitment to my Co-worker©

As your co-worker with a shared goal of providing excellent service to our clients, I commit to the following:

- I will accept responsibility for establishing and maintaining healthy interpersonal relationships with you and every member of this staff. I will talk to you promptly if I am having a problem with you. The only time I will discuss it with another person is when I need advice or help in deciding how to communicate with you appropriately
- I will establish and maintain functional trust with you and every other member of this staff. My relationships with each of you will be equally respectful, regardless of job titles or levels of educational preparation
- I will not engage in the *3 B's* (bickering, backbiting and blaming) and will ask you not to as well
- I will not complain about another team member, and ask you not to as well. If I hear you doing so, I will ask you to talk to that person
- I will accept you as you are today, forgiving past problems and ask you to do the same

continued

- I will be committed to finding solutions to problems rather than complaining about them or blaming someone for them and ask you to do the same with me
- I will affirm your contribution to the quality of our service
- I will remember that neither of us is perfect and that human errors are opportunities, not for shame and guilt but for forgiveness and growth

(compiled by Marie Manthey, 2003 © Creative Health Care Management)

Reflective activity

Think about the team in which you currently work.

- To what extent does your team meet the 'Commitment to my co-workers'? Identify how you are affected by the 'norms' being used in the team – can you identify examples of how you have unconsciously contributed to sustaining unhealthy behaviours?
- How can you change your behaviour to begin a positive change in the emotional intelligence of the team?

Senge (1990) celebrates proactivity thus:

> This is the true joy in life, the being used for a purpose recognised by yourself as a mighty one . . . the being a force of nature instead of a feverish, selfish little clod of ailments and grievances complaining that the world will not devote itself to making you happy.
>
> Shaw (1903), cited in Senge (1990, p. 352)

Having looked at what the essential behaviours are that we need in teams, we will go on to consider development.

Structured guidance on team development

In order to respect the differences that there are in teams, it is necessary to recognise not only those differences but also commonalities. There will be cultural differences, different ways of doing things and different behaviours that are acceptable in the workplace and in friendships. We do not often expect these if we assume that the person we are working with has similar experiences to us, and it can be a shock when we discover that our assumptions are wrong. It is useful to be specific and check out that the other person understands what you mean.

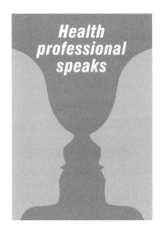

Health professional speaks

Member of a multi-professional team

It was very embarrassing. I asked her to help Mr Smith have a shave. The gentleman's family were so upset: he had worn a moustache for 60 years. I really didn't think I needed to say to only do the bits he usually does, I mean, she did as I asked, I suppose.

Reflective activity

Have you ever been in a meeting where you did not understand an abbreviation or a term being used? Did you ask?

If you do ask, you will be surprised how many people are pleased and also admit that they did not understand either!

The search for the Holy Grail

There is not one right answer that will sort everything out: it is not just that one person with whom you have a problem, or that changing this one thing will bring the success that you are looking for.

There is a difference between complicated and complex. When something is complex, there are too many variables for it ever to be truly known or fully understood, or managed. Life is complex. Organisations are complex (Allee, 2003, p. 61). We try to manage a situation by breaking it down into manageable parts, but parts work together in such a way that the situation cannot be divided without losing integrity (Allee, 2003, p. 62). We cannot manage it directly; we must each play our part as individuals managing our roles, our activities, our relationships and how we participate (Allee, 2003, p. 64).

Learning to work with complexity will require more than changing what we do; it will also require changing the way we think (Allee, 2003, p. 63).

No one person can understand; we need multiple lenses and minds. Together, we can seek meaningful patterns that help us to understand and take effective action (Allee, 2003, p. 63).

Change is not easy, even when we have accepted the need. People are not just minds: they are not only rational but also emotional and have emotional investments in the past and the present (Oshry, 1996, p. 199).

It is through building relationships and learning to question what we do with kindness and genuine care for our team members, and patients, that we can find solutions together. Do not leave it to someone else; you cannot do it on your own but there has to be a start somewhere.

Do not give up; remember that the greater the investment in the past, the louder the resistance or 'sounds of the old dance shaking'. When we step back and understand we are in a system and see its process, we can choose. No longer are we trapped by the system or by our politics. We can develop, respect and encourage our individuality, our community, our diversity and our commonality (Oshry, 1996, pp. 200–201).

RRRRR**Rapid recap**

Check your progress so far by working through each of the following questions.

1. List three characteristics of a team.
2. Identify and describe four types of groups or teams.
3. List the five leadership strategies of the CLIMB model.
4. What are the competencies displayed by successful teams?
5. What are the behaviours that you should exhibit when your team is less successful?

If you have difficulty with more than one of the questions, read through the section again to refresh your understanding before moving on.

References

Allee, V. (2003) *The Future of Knowledge: Increasing Prosperity through Value Networks*. Butterworth-Heinemann, Burlington MA.

Allen, M. and Pickering, C. (2002) *Core Competencies of Clinical Teams: Final Report*. The Deanery, University of Leeds, Leeds.

Bate, P. (1995) *Strategies for Cultural* Change. Butterworth-Heinemann, Oxford.

Bergmann, H., Hurson, K. and Russ-Eft, D. (1999) *Everyone a Leader: A Grassroots Model for the New Workplace*. John Wiley and Sons Inc., New York.

Borrill, C.S., Carletta, J., Carter, A., Dawson, J.F., Garrod, S., Rees, A., Richards, A., Shapiro, D. and West, M. (2002) *The Effectiveness of Health Care Teams in the National Health Service*. Aston Centre for Health Service Organisation Research, Birmingham: Aston Business School, University of Aston.

Buchanan, D. and Huczynski, A. (2004) *Organisational Behaviour: An Introductory Text*, 5th edn. Pearson Education Ltd., Harlow.

Covey, S. (1989) *The Seven Habits of Highly Effective People*. Simon and Schuster, New York.

Covey, S. (1992) *Principle-centred Leadership*. Simon and Schuster, London.

Creative Healthcare Management (2003) *Leading an Empowered Organisation: Training Manual*. CHCM, Minneapolis.

Goleman, D., Boyatzis, R. and Mckee, A. (2003) *The New Leaders: Transforming the Art of Leadership into the Science of Results*. Time Warner Paperbacks, London.

Halligan, A. (2003) The Implementation of Clinical Governance. *Health Director*, (Mar/Apr):14–15. www.cgsupport.nhs.uk/PDFs/articles/implementation_of_cg.pdf.

Johnson, G. and Scholes, K. (2002) *Exploring Corporate Strategy: Text and* Cases, 6th edn. Pearson Education, Harlow.

Katzenbach, J.R. and Smith, D.K. (1993) *The Wisdom of Teams: Creating the High Performance Organisation*. McGraw-Hill Publishing Company, Maidenhead.

Oshry, B. (1996) *Seeing Systems: Unlocking the Mysteries of Organisational Life*, paperback edn. Berret-Koehler Publishers, San Francisco.

Peters, T. and Waterman, R.H. (eds.) (2004) *In Search of Excellence*. Profile Books, London.

Reeves, T. (1998) *Alchemy for Managers: Turning Experience into Achievement*, revised edn. Butterworth-Heinemann, Oxford.

Senge, P.M. (1990) *The Fifth Discipline: The Art and Practice of the Learning Organisation*. Random House, London.

Walshe, K. and Higgins, J. (2002) The Use and Impact of Inquiries in the NHS. *BMJ*, **325**(19 Oct.): 895–900

West, M.A. and Markiewicz, L. (2004) *Building Team Based Working: A Practical Guide to Organisational Transformation*. Blackwell, Oxford.

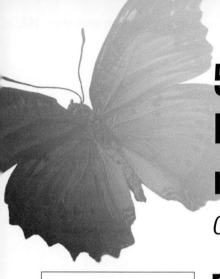

5
Effective team management

Chris White

Learning outcomes

By the end of this chapter you should be able to:

★ Understand management practice in the context of its origins

★ Explain different roles in teams

★ Be able to recognise and use communication and feedback

★ Understand your team in the context of a system

★ Have a working knowledge of techniques to help teams

★ Explain transition.

Overview of the theory

> The Japanese are famous for teamwork; they naturally do things in groups or teams. We in the Anglo-Saxon world do not share this same desire to be in groups, our culture rewards and values individual effort. No matter how much teamwork achieves, the results tend to be attributed to a single name.
>
> Furnham (cited in Billsberry, 1996, p. 179)

Reeves (1998, p. 10) defines management as working through other people to achieve a purpose or goal, whether or not you would describe yourself as a manager. By this definition, most people manage something in health care organisations, for example shifts, smaller teams looking after specific patient areas, specialities within larger teams, delegating to assistants, or responsibility for and audit of an aspect of care.

The beginnings of management practice come from bureaucratic and military models, which have defined the practices that have become common (Allee, 2003, p. 6).

What are we managing?

Effectiveness is about getting results and must be defined for each situation because of the unique interaction between the people and the circumstances (Reeves, 1998, p. 12).

The results are our progress to where we need to be in order to meet the demands of users, targets, standards and research (quality), capacity (amount of demand), both now and when planning to continue to meet these changing demands in the future.

Resources

The skills that we use in organising our personal lives are used in the workplace but on a bigger scale. Making sure that the budget lasts and necessary supplies are provided is not essentially different from personal budgeting for food, clothes and holidays, for example. The mystery that traditionally surrounds departmental budgets is a symptom of knowledge being used as power. For team members to own and take responsibility for aspects of service delivery in daily practice, information must be shared. It is a myth that front-line workers do not need to concern themselves with these things. Large organisations are particularly prone to waste because repetition occurs in different parts without anyone noticing.

One of the reasons that people keep their heads down and avoid knowing about difficult things is that it is easier to moan that resources are always allocated somewhere else than to try to understand the priorities and pressures of the organisation and to work with them to your advantage.

Performance

Clinical performance also needs managing because it is all too easy to be so busy with your own caseload that you repeat lessons already learnt, become isolated from peers and therefore do not use them as a resource for checking out decisions and standardised practice. There are many ways of measuring and checking our performance as individuals and as teams: audit against standards and guidelines, benchmarking and comparisons in capacity and quality.

Development

Benchmarking where we are at a point in time is only the beginning. The information that we have on how we are doing today informs the plans for tomorrow, and each of us has a part to play in working towards better services for the future. Sometimes we can refine what we are already doing to better effect, and sometimes a major overhaul is required, which can be shocking and unsettling.

Effectiveness

The areas of effectiveness are:

- safety
- clinical and cost effectiveness
- governance
- patient focus
- accessible and responsive care
- care environment and amenities
- public health
  (DoH, 2006).

Evidence base

Read Department of Health (2006) *Standards for Better Health*, with particular reference to the Core and Developmental Standards – pages 10–17 (www.dh.gov.uk/publications).

Everyone who is working effectively contributes to these areas of work. For example:

- **Safety**. Equipment should be checked to see that it is in good working order before use. Incidents and accidents should be reported so that trends are noticed. Regulations should be observed, for example, in relation to fire safety. Unnecessary risks should not be taken.

- **Clinical and cost effectiveness**. There should be wise use of resources including time, and awareness of cost in terms of finance and best value (for example a wound dressing that is more expensive may be cost effective if healing will be accelerated so less will be used). Each team member should contribute to staying within the allocated budget. There should be understanding of the impact of sickness in terms of team effectiveness and finances. Practice is evidence based, evaluated and audited.

- **Governance**. There should be accountability throughout organisations in all aspects of leading and managing, so that systems of working give, and improve, quality and safety. This means that the culture of development encourages suggestions and comments from staff and patients.

- **Patient focus**. There should be respect and partnership with patients and with other agencies for the patient's benefit, keeping the whole patient journey in mind and not abdicating responsibility for other parts if the patient needs help or advice.

- **Accessible and responsive care**. Choice should be given and unnecessary delays avoided in relation to services and treatments.

- **Care environment and amenities**. There should be suitably designed and maintained facilities for staff wellbeing and to respect patients' needs, preferences and privacy.

- **Public health**. Not only should preventative advice be given to individuals but practitioners should think in terms of communities and challenge systems that disadvantage groups or individuals, and collaborate with other organisations.

What is important about having standards is avoiding the pitfall of targets that focus attention and resources into some areas at the expense of others; a rounded approach, as attempted in the document referred to in the evidence base feature on page 105, seeks to keep attention on all areas at once.

If performance is not measured against standards, it is not possible to be objective about how you are doing. Other perspectives such as staff and patient surveys clearly have uses but are essentially subjective, and there is the danger that expectations may be too low or too high. Such surveys need to be taken into account when considering standards, not used instead of them.

○━ᴨ *Keywords*

SMART objectives
Are specific objectives that
are set out in such a way
that it is clear who is doing
what and by when; SMART
is an acronym for:
Specific
Measurable
Achievable
Realistic
Timebound

Shared responsibility helps to keep a focus on the big picture and tends to cascade knowledge and accountability for what is required to teams. These can be translated into what is required of teams and individuals by setting **SMART objectives** in service areas, and translating these to personal development plans.

This makes sure that the objective is 'owned' by everyone and avoids the trap of 'leaving it to someone else'.

Thinking of management as getting things done through others recognises that all of us manage in some form. It is important to consider how we will know if what we do personally is effective in contributing to the standard. This really comes down to behaviours. There are three ways to think about being effective:

- what you put into an activity or task

- the process you use in your work

- what contribution this makes to personal and team objectives (Reeves, 1998, pp. 21–22).

Interconnectedness

Each member of a team makes a unique contribution. You will have experienced this when working shifts with different people: the workplace can feel quite different when someone is either there or not there. We each bring our personal qualities: enthusiasm, sociability, persuasion, imagination, lateral thinking, knowledge and experience, motivation, commitment, **empathy**, taking responsibility for decisions, willingness to do mundane tasks, and the ability to carry on when things do not go according to plan (Reeves, 1998, p. 35).

○━ᴨ *Keywords*

Empathy
Is the ability to understand
and share the feelings of
another

Reflective activity

The person you are and your attitudes affect the way that others around you work and perform, and how they are affects your work and performance.

- Can you identify a handover or staff meeting when your reaction to a topic or delegated task was a direct result of someone else's behaviour or attitude? Were others affected? How could this have been handled differently?

- If your reaction was counter-productive, identify how you would behave differently before and/or during a similar meeting. List the positive effects that this would have on the emotions of staff and on patient care during that shift.

Roles within a team

Within teams, some roles are given as part of a job description that allocates responsibility for certain aspects of care and performance. Other roles are taken because of a person's individual personality, skills or experience and are equally important to efficient team function. In the late 1970s, Belbin and colleagues developed the following framework for understanding roles within teams. It describes nine roles:

- plant – creates imaginative ideas, proposes novel solutions to difficult problems, prefers to work alone, sensitive to praise and criticism
- resource-investigator – good communicator, enthusiastic, extrovert, likes networking, good at negotiation, easily bored
- coordinator – good chairperson, delegates well, clarifies and promotes decision making; good at recognising an individual's abilities and getting them involved; keeps the group on track towards the objective
- shaper – highly motivated, thrives on pressure, challenging, needs to achieve; can appear pushy and aggressive
- monitor-evaluator – steady, not displaying excesses of emotion, strategic and serious; sees the options and critically judges slowly but accurately
- teamworker – diplomatic and cooperative; provides support for others in the team; avoids conflict and allows others to contribute to the task
- implementer – efficient, practical, reliable; likes routine and being systematic
- completer – conscientious, gives attention to detail, anxious; relies on themselves and delivers on time with high standards
- specialist – has specific technical skill, focused, dedicated; more interested in their professional standards than in the team's work and its members.

(Buchanan and Huczynski, 2004, p. 336)

Reflective activity

No one takes on only one role. In your team, decide which two or three roles you each take most regularly. As a team, think what roles are needed for what you are doing at the moment and if there are roles missing from the members' top three preferred roles (Buchanan and Huczynski, 2004, pp. 337 and 350).

- What is the impact on patient care of these missing roles? Is every shift affected?
- If there is a mismatch, for example more than one specialist in the same area in a shift, what can be done to organise the spread differently?
- Are there other roles that should be spread or are some team members more effective when they work together? Why is this?
- What about non-clinical tasks such as administration?

Essential team management behaviours

We have looked at practical necessities for managing resources, at using evidence and measuring where we are to enable development planning, and at how these aspects are essential for those with a job title that includes the word 'manager', and for everyone else in the team too.

It is essential to have systems and processes in place that prevent waste. Waste can occur when learning or duties have to be repeated because of lack of information; when there is spending on items that are not used to full effect; and when there is short-term thinking, such as using cheaper items that are not as effective so that more are used, which costs more in the long run.

Even when good systems and processes are in place, these rely on people to make them work; this can be said of our clinical interactions as well as interactions in or across teams. We will now look at behaviours that make or break systems.

Communication

There are many different types of communication that are used for different purposes. Non-verbal communication, also known as body language, tells others a lot about what we are thinking and feeling without the need for words. 'Actions speak louder than words' is a common saying when a person does not match their behaviour to what they say (Improvement Leaders Guides, 2005a, p. 33).

The term 'poor communication' is not very helpful as there may be different expectations of the giver and receiver as well as differences of opinion about what it is essential to know and what the person would like to know (Honey, 2001, p. 41).

The best technology infrastructure for sharing information, for example websites, emails, text messages and voicemail, cannot overcome other cultural and structural barriers such as mistrust and internal competition. Improving the intelligence in an organisation is not a technological question: it is a human question (Allee, 2003, p. 89).

It is not difficult to send out information; before we had access to technology we used notice boards, but hardly anyone looked at them. The same is true of any form of information sharing; the point is that giving information is not communication. Communication involves confirming that the message you intended to give was heard and understood in the way that you meant it by checking out what the recipient thinks you said. You should also understand how they feel about what you said and if, the communication concerned an action, check if anything further needs to be done to enable that action to happen.

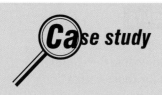

Case study

Contrasting styles of team leader communication

A highly technical team leader avoided contact with the team by communicating all the time by emails, with the effect that team members became disengaged. In contrast, a team leader with excellent people skills avoided communicating difficult issues about performance by email.

- What kinds of communication are appropriate by email and which are not?
- How is it best to communicate difficult issues?
- Why is this not only important for those with the title 'leader' but also for other people?

It is important to take responsibility for communication, whatever your job title. If you think that there is something that you should know, then ask; do not wait for someone to seek you out.

We need general information in our workplace to understand the context of what we are doing and how it fits with the organisation, but the most important form of communication that we need, as individuals and as teams, is feedback: to know if what we are doing is appropriate, and to be able to adjust what we do so that it continues to be right in the light of changes around us. We adapt to what an individual prefers or needs, but it is important to check out if our assumptions are right.

What is feedback?

It is not possible to learn or maintain good performance without feedback, but there are several reasons why teams lack it:

- There may be a culture of avoiding receiving feedback because of fear of criticism.
- Team members may avoid giving feedback within the team because they do not want to upset the other person.
- Individuals may lack the skills to receive feedback in a way that leads to learning.
- Members and leaders may lack the skill to be constructive so that the people become disillusioned instead of encouraged to action (Honey 2001, p. 72).

Goleman *et al.* (2003, p. 168) agree, describing fear of the leader's wrath, not wanting to bring bad news and wanting to be a team player as the phenomena that make people deny their leader's essential feedback. Honest, helpful feedback can be difficult to give when there is a culture of compliance because of fear of punishment for stepping out of line.

Cultures that promote useful feedback take time to evolve because they are dependent on building relationships, and this does not happen overnight. If you are in this situation, build a relationship by seeking feedback for yourself first, and give feedback with regard to what you are learning from what you were told and how it is helping your practice to develop.

In time, when the benefits are seen, others will begin to question themselves and start to seek feedback – start gently and be positive.

Punitive feedback is sadly more common than positive feedback despite the greater likelihood that people will do things right rather than wrong. Negative feedback is counter-productive as it leads to the opposite of the desired effect, which is the open-minded, non-defensive receipt of feedback that leads to learning and results in a specific action plan for improvements (Honey, 2001, p. 72). Open and honest discussions are essential in teams for sharing the pressures of work and understanding what individual team members need.

Feedback on performance can reveal previously unnoticed aspects of self or behaviour which, if fed back, can stimulate thinking and facilitate learning. It is usually the team member who observes your daily work who can give the most effective feedback (Reeves, 1997, p. 240).

✍ Over to you

Identify a person whom you work alongside and with whom you could build a mutual open and honest relationship in order to reflect and give each other feedback. Keep a journal of events for reflection that you can share.

Team reflection and journal club

The idea of a group of staff getting together, taking turns to read and present professional articles is not new. Often, this takes place within our professions rather than in teams because we dislike it when others challenge our perspective or ask obvious questions. We tell ourselves that they do not understand. Actually, they do understand that we are entrenched in our perspectives (but maybe not that they are too!) and it would do us – and them – good if we were to get together and willingly seek challenge that would stimulate us to explore our own thinking.

We need to become aware of how what we say and do is influenced by our underlying assumptions and **mental models**. New experiences that conflict with our beliefs are not recognised because they do not fit with our model, causing inconsistencies in what we believe, say and do. (See page 113 for discussion of how mental models affect team behaviours.)

Looking at evidence from other disciplines that share our patients' journeys will help us to uncover ideas that need to be challenged as we learn the skills of what Senge (1990, p. 278) calls 'participative openness'. These skills take persistence and time, since it is necessary to inquire, reflect and suspend judgement in dialogue (Senge, 1990,

🗝 Keywords

Mental model
Is a way of making sense of things by building on deeply ingrained patterns of thinking and assumptions from previous experience

p. 278).

Seeing how our actions may be creating the very problems that we are trying to resolve means that we must think about the whole system, not just our part, and learn from it (Senge, 1990, p. 238).

Systems thinking (seeing the bigger picture)

Senge (1990, p. 6) uses the illustration of a storm gathering to show how we build up connections among sometimes seemingly unconnected events to understand patterns. Although a time delay between some events may, in some cases, make it difficult for us to see the connections, the individual events do not make sense on their own. It can take years for the interrelations and their consequences to become apparent and, as we are part of our systems, it is very hard to see the whole or to accept that our own actions and behaviours actually contribute to the problems that we are experiencing.

The principle of understanding the whole system applies to teams in three ways:

- how our contribution fits into the team's purpose
- the way our team fits with the system through the patient's journey
- the bigger picture.

In addition, we need to be aware of how our work contributes to the team's purpose and how that positively affects the whole team, and thus the patient's experience, when we are functioning at optimum. Also important is awareness of the effects on the team and patients when we are not functioning well.

In good teams, performance is smoothed out – we help each other. However, if we could look deeper and think about the conditions that contribute to good days, we might be able to do more to foster those conditions and have more good days, thus providing a better service and enjoying our work, and having some fun and feeling a sense of achievement into the bargain.

Everyone must have some experience of trying to get through on the telephone to someone who can answer a question and being passed from department to department, with no one willing to take the initiative and responsibility for resolving the problem. If we could truly look at what we are doing from the perspective of the individual patient, then, at the very minimum, we would want to understand fully what happens before and after our contribution. Then we could smooth the process in relation to how we receive patients and refer them on, knowing how important the little things are: for example a personal introduction, a smile, a welcome – common courtesies that help people to feel at ease and be at their best too.

The bigger picture is very relative to where you are, whether within a department or division. It could relate to the organisation as a whole, or the position that the organisation holds within the health and social care system or community in which you are situated. It could involve policy decisions at a local or national level. In fact, everything is part of some system, and the impact of the influences overlap, for example cultural differences, which can change the way that other elements are perceived.

It is important to realise that what you do either upholds or undermines what is happening with the bigger picture. So you need to know at least something about that picture and choose your behaviours appropriately.

Reflective activity

Take it upon yourself, while you are with patients, to ask them individually about their current experience. Ask if they can tell you one thing that works well and also suggest one area for improvement.

Don't try to defend the system but think about it from their point of view. How can you do more of the good thing? Who could implement the suggested improvement? Can you do it? Can your team do it? Is the problem at more than one point in the system? Can you make it your business to influence that?

Insidious problems

Senge (1990, p. 22) tells the 'boiled frog' parable to alert us to the danger of slowly developing problems. If a frog is placed in a pot of hot water, it will jump out. However, if a frog is placed in cool water and heated slowly, it will not notice the change and it will happily sit there and boil. We need to step back and look for gradually creeping problems to avoid the same fate.

It can be difficult to learn from experience, which is the way we learn best, when we do not directly experience the consequences that we cause (Senge, 1990, p. 23). We have to go and look for these.

Structured reflection on team behaviours

Before we go on to explore some practical ways of developing team behaviours, let's look first at what they are.

Mental models

Have you ever learnt something new, suddenly had an insight, or been told something that you have tried and found to be true but just not been able to change your habits so as to keep doing it?

This happens in management; even new ideas that have been tried and tested on a small scale and have been shown to work in the environment fail to become standard practice because of the way that we think. As we saw previously, we have deeply ingrained patterns of thinking and assumptions, of which we are probably not even aware, that may conflict with new ideas causing us to reject them. It takes discipline to examine these foundations, uncover and scrutinise them, learning the balance between advocating our views and, seeking to learn, listening to the views of others (Senge, 1990, p. 8).

Sharing vision

In any kind of organisation, success in fulfilling its purpose or meeting its goal is dependent on each member working towards that purpose. This is not because there is a 'vision statement' on the wall, but because each person has an understanding of principles and practices that work towards a common identity. Building a vision that is shared from individual visions fosters genuine commitment with people wanting to excel and learn (Senge, 1990, p. 9).

Meetings

Meetings can have a reputation for not being 'proper work', perhaps because they can be non-productive. There are several possible reasons for this: the wrong people present, for example people who are unable to make the necessary commitments; sidetracking; lack of purpose; interruptions; not making decisions; and long, over-ambitious agendas (Honey, 2001, p. 124).

It is essential to keep in mind the purposes of the meeting, breaking these down by agenda items and distinguishing between information sharing and seeking decisions. Creating new possibilities or choosing from a limited range of options, giving advice, or being asked to find resources are common reasons to meet, and it is important to understand what is expected of you.

Reflective activity

Prepare for the next team meeting by finding out what is on the agenda and thinking through your perspective on it. Will you be representing or advocating the views of other staff or patients, and do you need to seek their opinions to check out assumptions? Is there any information or evidence that you can take with you?

'Them' and 'us'

Front-line workers often form into a 'we' that excludes others, pressurising 'members' to conform. Those who do not conform are thrown out of the group. The 'we' leads to a feeling of 'them', and this can range from the mild, such as a laugh at the expense of the supervisor, to the more serious, such as breaking 'their' rules, sabotage, and so on. Maintenance of the 'we' group relies on members' not admitting differences, to others and sometimes to themselves. On occasions, people do openly disagree but are ignored by the group, being treated as 'village idiots' (Oshry, 1996, p. 135).

Thinking in terms of 'them' and 'us' is an unhelpful way to behave because it tends to ignore that we are all individually responsible for our own actions and behaviours and the effect that these have on our colleagues. It also makes it easier to justify feelings that may be caused by misunderstanding, or not having enough information to understand the whole story, and may lead to a vicious cycle of feeling badly done to, when others reinforce this.

We need to promote and understand different perspectives that provide us with insights, learning to question each other in a supportive way.

Structured guidance on team development

Having looked at common team behaviours, we now consider practical ways to develop teams by promoting effectiveness, working together and helpful behaviours.

Improving meeting performance

- **Plan.** Arrange dates and send out agendas and items for discussion in advance. Allocate time for each agenda item by agreement at the beginning of the meeting and agree adjustments accordingly if there is not enough time for all the items.
- **Time.** Start and finish on time, agree necessary changes – don't just allow items to overrun.
- **Accountability.** Capture actions, identifying who will do what and by when clearly for each point and highlight in the minutes. Distribute meeting minutes promptly as a reminder.
- **People.** Share good news, be open and honest about things that need attention but make positive plans to tackle these, finish on positives. The 'glue' of teams is relationships, so plan occasional social events.
- **Clarify** Ask if you are not sure about something so as to avoid wasted time and effort.

Process mapping

Process mapping is a powerful yet simple way to combine thinking about the whole system and the service users' perspective. It points out 'handoffs' (that is, the number of times that the 'job' is passed from one person or department to another person or department) and delays: for example, having been seen by a doctor, patients wait for tests. Getting all the professions together allows questions from different perspectives that challenge why the system is how it is, and this, in itself, can lead to finding a better way to do something.

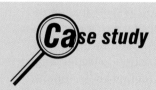

Case study

Changing the way systems work

The team looked at the way that equipment repairs – mainly to hoists and wheelchairs – were carried out. Such repairs should be done urgently because these pieces of equipment are used all the time in people's homes. The team realised that handoffs were causing delays. They decided that if they emailed the request to the subcontractor, they would save a lot of time and the subcontractor would be able to log the request when it was received, enabling the team to check that each request was being dealt with.

The team members were able to analyse why they did things in certain ways. Sometimes, it was just for historical reasons: there was no rationale; it had always been done that way. As they were working together, they were able to challenge the reasons for certain procedures, and they were able to agree that the patient could call the repairer directly for some repairs. This was a much more responsive way of doing things. It was not rocket science, but the team had never looked at the whole picture.

- Are you aware of the issues that your patients have?
- Who needs to be round the table to map that process?

Double-loop learning

Argyris and Schon (in Revans, 1998) described single- and double-loop learning. In single-loop learning, performance is maintained (like a thermostat), and it never questions the norm. Double-loop learning challenges assumptions, beliefs, norms, routines and decisions, asking the question, 'Is that target appropriate?'

Process mapping is a really good way to get everyone involved because they know how it works and contribute their ideas. Together, they can see parts that can be improved and take ownership for the whole, whereas, previously, everyone felt that other parts had nothing to do with them.

Mapping a process

It is important to involve the right people – clinicians and managers – for the process that you are looking at, and these people should be included from the start, thus ensuring their support for putting into practice any recommended changes. Ideally, there should be 15–20 staff, representing all the stages of the patient journey, to promote lots of discussion. The venue you choose must be suitable to encourage attendance and participation, and, as people will have to arrange cover for their work, they will need plenty of notice (Improvement Leaders Guides, 2005b, pp. 12–13).

Write all the stages of the journey on Post-it notes so that you can move them around as you identify other stages; then rearrange them in a branching map-like configuration to show concurrent events. Avoid the temptation to start solving problems before you have the whole process mapped!

Put the configuration on a wall where everyone can see it and contribute. Decide how you are going to generate ideas from it, and discuss these with the service manager and lead clinician (Improvement Leaders Guides, 2005b, p. 15). Make the process fun and celebratory so as to maximise the team-building effect: the greater the involvement at this stage, the more commitment there will be to the improvement effort that the team decides on.

Test it out

Try to get people involved: start with something quite small so that you can demonstrate a positive result fairly quickly; experiment with ideas; look for the evidence; try things out; evaluate. Be positive even if an idea doesn't work; at least you know that now, and you tried it on a small scale. Be proactive and try several things at once in small groups; do not only look for one right answer. When people have been involved in something small that they can see has worked, they will be less frightened of change.

Plan, Do, Study, Act

This is a good way to test an idea:

- **Plan**. Agree what is to be tested – set objectives, ask questions – Who? What? Where? When? – and plan what data collection you will need, before and after the change to answer these questions.

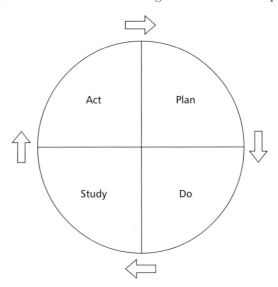

The PDSA cycle to test a change idea (adapted from Improvement Leaders Guides, 2005b, p. 24)

- **Do**. Collect the 'before' data; carry out the change and measure the impact by collecting the 'after' data.
- **Study**. Analyse the data; compare with what you expected to find; summarise what you learnt. Is the change an improvement?
- **Act**. Plan the next change cycle or implementation of the idea.

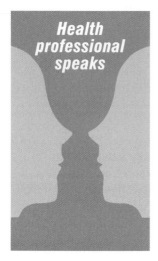

Health professional speaks

Team leader

All of my work is projects, reporting each to the person taking corporate responsibility for that area. Some are within our department, some across the division, and some are corporate, reporting to the board and to others across organisations.

This sounds complicated, but the principle is simple: the boundaries that we perceive are actually not real for the patients who use the services; projects are organised through the journey that the patient takes, smoothing out the block-ages and delays in the system. Networks are built up that help to sort out problems. It is easier to work for solutions when the right people are working together across the health and social care community for the same overall aim. It means that I can work it out rather than passing it on to my line manager, who passes it on again until it crosses to another organisation and then comes down their chain of command, like things used to be. Now, I can just keep my manager informed and get on with finding out whom I need to speak with to sort it out.

Reflective activity

- Identify the ways in which this team leader is taking responsibility.
- Why is it important to keep others informed when working in this way?

Project management

The most commonly cited reason for why change projects fail is neglecting the human parts of the process, not managing why people are unhappy with change, not understanding the change process and not using the techniques that are available to help.

Both approaches to improvement are needed.

The commitment of people who will be affected by the change is essential; without this the improvement project will be hampered because:

- There are strong emotions of fear, anger, frustration and hopelessness.

Table 5.1 Approaches to improvement

Concentrating on one part at a time	Thinking about the whole	Reasons why both approaches are necessary
Change is a step-by-step process	Outcomes cannot be predetermined	You need to set a direction but need to be flexible
It is typically initiated top down	Actual change comes typically bottom up	Top-down support is needed for bottom-up change
Objectives set in advance (and set in stone!)	There is no end point	Objectives need to be set and the team should be congratulated when each objective is achieved but improvement never ends
It goes wrong because of poor planning and project control	It goes wrong because of people issues	Planning and monitoring is important but gaining the commitment of people is vital

(adapted from Improvement Leaders Guides, 2005a)

- There is defensiveness, blaming others; people become unrealistic about what they are doing now and about the proposed change.
- There is often scepticism, complaining and constant questioning.
- There may be low morale with an increase in sickness, absenteeism and staff leaving.
- People do not do what they say they are going to do.
- Conflict seems to be out of control.

(Improvement Leaders Guides, 2005a)

Change: unfreezing and refreezing

Joseph Raelin presents a useful discussion of the ideas of Kurt Lewin. A change challenges the status quo, known as 'unfreezing'; there is then a state of change before the new way of doing things is established, 'refreezing' (Raelin, 2003, pp. 158 and 163).

There are forces for change and forces for stability (against change); these can be mapped and their strength estimated. If forces for change are strengthened without decreasing forces against, this can cause more resistance. Lewin advised identifying and lessening forces against, so that the balance changes rather than increasing forces for change (Raelin, 2003, p. 159).

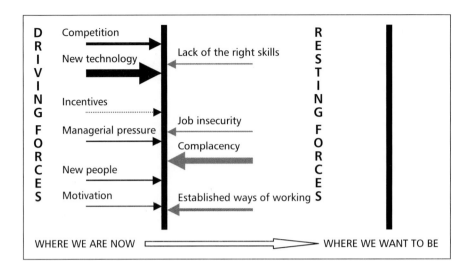

Lewin's Force Field model (adapted from Iles & Sutherland, 2001, p. 44)

Over to you

With your team, construct a force field analysis for a change. Draw arrows facing a central line. How big an arrow should each issue have based on the strength of the force? What are the positive factors for change? What are the factors supporting staying as things are? What can be done to influence these factors? Who else cares about the issue and can help? What behaviours will you need to contribute and influence?

An additional project management framework that you are likely to encounter as your career progresses is Prince 2®. This involves the use of a specific, structured approach to the organisation, management and control of large or complex projects. Additional information is available through the website: www.ogc.gov.uk/prince2.

Continuous quality improvement

Also known as total quality management, this sums up the idea that we must constantly be aware of changes and adapt accordingly. There are four principles:

- For an organisation to be successful, each department has to be meeting the needs of the service users.
- The processes of production are what cause quality in a complex but understandable system.

- Most people are motivated from within themselves to work hard and to do well.
- The use of data and simple analysis give powerful insights into problems with the work processes.

(Iles and Sutherland, 2001, p. 48)

On a day-to-day basis, people don't notice that some areas of practice that should be challenged because they have always been done that way. Using data will also help teams to know what the distant effects of their work are and work towards better quality throughout the patient journey, not just the parts that they can see in the here and now.

Usually, data collection requires the people doing the work to collect and input the data and, at this point, it can be difficult to see the benefit, especially if that part of the process encroaches on time that could be spent with patients. It is worth asking what the data are used for and ensuring that the reports that are produced can be shared with the team. It is useful to decide what it is that your team would like to know to help to improve the quality and efficiency of the service and to see if the data have already been collected in some form or could more usefully be collected than something already monitored.

Solution focus

We spend a lot of time and emotional energy looking at problems in health care. This can promote negative thoughts and drain enthusiasm by making us feel guilty.

Focusing on solutions and on doing more of what works engenders a positive mindset and promotes improvement in small manageable steps. Although solution focus can be used as a psychological intervention, it does not require expert knowledge because it relies on allowing people to identify their own solutions by asking specific and positive questions.

Quite simply, solution focus involves:

- acknowledging the problem – how is it a problem to you?
- defining how you would like the future to be
- finding out what helps to make progress towards this future
- doing more of what works
- if something doesn't work, stopping and doing something else.

The future is described by asking 'the miracle question', that is, asking how you would know if a miracle had happened and this problem had gone. Visualise in detail life without this problem. What has changed? Who else notices?

To see what helps, ask about occasions when the problem has been less or about other situations when the problem does not occur. What circumstances and behaviours make it less? More of these will facilitate progress towards the goal.

To visualise progress, use a scale of 0–10, where 0 is the problem at its worst and 10 is the vision of the future. Ask where you are at the moment on this scale, being positive about any progress towards the goal that has already been achieved. Visualise what one step nearer would be like. Taking small steps is essential because they are achievable and often start a positive chain of events.

During questioning it is important to be positive, looking for opportunities to compliment, either directly, such as 'You handled that brilliantly!', or indirectly, such as 'How did you manage to do such a difficult task?' These indicate resources and solutions that the person already has and help to identify what works (Visser and Bodien, no date).

The person is to decide what works, based on previous success that they have forgotten about because of focusing on problems instead of solutions. This increases both confidence and commitment to try proposed solutions, and, as small steps in the right direction are what are intended, the risk of the solution's not working is lessened.

Reflective activity

Choose a current problem and practise solution-focused problem solving with someone. You will be surprised how difficult it is, at first, to stay positive and not to give advice! It is worth the practice because visualising and focusing on what you know you can already do is amazingly motivating for both of you.

Managing conflict

There is a huge range of behaviours that might be considered conflict, from minor disagreements to outright attempts to destroy each other. Conflict needs to be managed because it is a reality and can be turned around to positive ends. It is important that conflict is sorted out as soon as possible because of the adverse effect that it has on the people concerned and on the rest of the team. There is nothing more wearing than a constant 'atmosphere' and getting caught up in disagreements. As well as the original issues, the breakdown in relationship between the people concerned also becomes a problem (Improvement Leaders Guides, 2005a, p. 29).

All of us know from personal experiences that the longer bad feelings are left to fester, the harder they are to sort out. It is useful to clarify what the purpose of a challenge is because what seems like conflict may not be. Challenging ideas is not wrong: it may only be that it is being done in an aggressive way; some people just enjoy a good argument. Some people also take any challenge as a personal criticism when none is intended.

There are three ways to deal with conflict in a team:

- preventing escalation – identifying early signs of hot (confrontational) or cold (silent seething) conflict and acting to prevent this worsening

Table 5.2 Handling conflict dos and don'ts

Do	Don't
• work to cool down the debate in a hot conflict	• talk in a public place
• convince parties in a cold conflict that something can be done	• leave the discussion open – agree next steps
• make sure that the issues are fully outlined by all	• finish the other person's sentence for them
• acknowledge emotions and different styles	• use jargon
• make sure you have a comfortable environment for any meeting	• constantly interrupt
• set a time frame for the discussion	• do something else whilst trying to listen
• ensure good rapport	• distort the truth
• use names and, if appropriate, titles throughout	• use inappropriate humour

(adapted from Improvement Leaders Guides, 2005a, p. 31)

- containing – dealing with difficulties by understanding and valuing the differences; seeking a solution that both can agree and working to restore relationships
- handling – dealing with conflict issues and monitoring them (Improvement Leaders Guides, 2005a, p. 30).

Managing transitions

Change is the new situation in which you find yourself; what causes the problem is the transition or psychological adjustment to that change. If change happens to us and we do not adjust, we go back to the old way when the dust settles. The transition starts with an ending, letting go of the old situation. This is the largest single problem with change management because it is often ignored. The next stage is between the old going and the new feeling comfortable – the neutral zone. This is an uncomfortable stage but offers a great opportunity for creativity and development, and should not be rushed. New habits form as things that no longer work in the situation are dropped. Then, the new beginning is when the new way feels comfortable and like the right way to do things (Bridges, 2002, p. 4).

Because we know from previous experience that change is painful, we may not tell people what is happening until the last minute. Or worse, there is sometimes no warning of change, and those concerned may only find out when the change starts, and we then ignore the pain and suffering that it causes, thinking that there was no point in doing it any differently because people will, in any case, be upset.

This is a great example of when leadership and management skills are needed together – combining the structure and planning of management with the people skills and empathy of leadership.

Grief

Overreaction is common: it may be a sign of grief, personal loss suffered as a result of the change, or a sign of previous hurt and an indication that grief processes from that occasion were never completely dealt with. It is much easier to be objective and reasonable if we have nothing at stake personally. If a small change is perceived as the start of something bigger that may affect others later, a similar reaction is understandable (Bridges, 2002, p. 23).

As in any other grief reaction, emotions may not show to begin with but all the recognised stages of grief are identified, starting with denial, which is followed by anger, bargaining or trying to get away from the situation, anxiety, sadness, disorientation and depression. Not every person goes through all the stages, but in a team all the stages will be experienced at one time or another – with individuals probably at different stages of the grief process, as everyone is different. What we need to think through is how we can compensate for what we feel we have lost, whether that is status, recognition or control over events (Bridges, 2002, p. 27).

It is really important to keep talking about the grief, and, at all stages, to allow feelings to be worked through, letting people know that they are listened to.

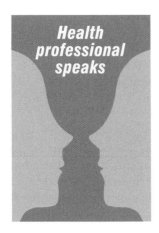

Health professional speaks

Physiotherapist

In a pain management team, the feedback we got from patients was that it was more important that someone listened to them and believed them than that we found a 'cure' or a solution to their pain. On reflection, I think we are probably all like that: we can understand that some things just won't go away, but, if we feel that someone cares, we can find the resources within ourselves to cope and move forward into planning for the future with optimism.

It is important to accept that loss is very subjective: what is a big issue to one person may mean nothing to others. Accept and acknowledge each other's losses and, without disputing how that feels, respect and value the past and people's contribution while being clear about what has and what has not ended (Improvement Leaders Guides, 2005a, p. 7).

Moving on

It is quite normal for human beings to respond to a shock or upset by denial until we cannot avoid the issue any longer. Next, comes anger; this is very stressful for all concerned, especially if it goes on too long, as it can cause physical illness. At this stage, everything feels uncertain and as if we are in an emotional fog; it doesn't make sense and we can't see a way out. The next stage is depression and despair, when we think that there will be no end to the situation. We want to be left alone or to seek others going through the same thing – who may be able to help.

The last stage is accepting what is happening. When the information starts to make some sense, we begin to see opportunities and new ideas and find ways of dealing with the situation. Whether we have chosen the change for ourselves or it has been forced on us, we must go through these stages to one degree or another before we can move on (Improvement Leaders Guides, 2005a, p. 9).

Ride the wave

It is much better to be proactive in change. I think of it like a huge wave coming in to the shore. You can run out to greet it and get on your surf board, experiencing exhilaration as well as fear, or you can sit on the beach and wait for it to crash over you, knowing only the fear.

RRRRRRapid recap

Check your progress so far by working through each of the following questions

1. How can effectiveness be defined?
2. What are the key areas that everyone is accountable for delivering to ensure effectiveness in health care?
3. What is the purpose of a SMART objective and what does the acronym stand for?
4. Name and describe four of the roles identified by Belbin that people adopt when working in teams.
5. How can you encourage an appropriate feedback culture in your team?
6. Identify five features of a solution-focused approach.

If you have difficulty with more than one of the questions, read through the section again to refresh your understanding before moving on.

References

Allee, V. (2003) *The Future of Knowledge: Increasing Prosperity through Value Networks*. Butterworth-Heinemann, Burlington MA.

Billsberry, J. (1996) *The Effective Manager: Perspectives and Illustrations*. SAGE Publications Ltd., London.

Bridges, W. (2002) *Managing Transitions: Making the Most of Change*, revised edn. Nicholas Brealey Publishing, London.

Buchanan, D. and Huczynski, A. (2004) *Organisational Behaviour: An Introductory Text*, 5th edn. Pearson Education Limited, Harlow.

Department of Health (2004) *Standards for Better Health*, updated 3 Apr. 2006. Gateway Reference updated version 6405, www.dh.gov.uk.

Department of Health (2006) *Standards for Better Health*. Department of Health Publications, PO Box 77, London.

Goleman, D., Boyatzis, R. and Mckee, A. (eds) (2003) *The New Leaders: Transforming the Art of Leadership into the Science of Results*. Time Warner Paperbacks, London.

Honey, P. (2001) *Improve Your People Skills*, revised 2nd edn. Chartered Institute of Personnel and Development, London.

Iles, V. and Sutherland, K. (2001) *Managing Change in the NHS, Organisational Change: A Review for Health Care Managers, Professionals and Researchers*. NCCSDO, London School of Hygiene and Tropical Medicine, London.

Improvement Leaders Guides (2005a) Gateway reference 4701. *Managing the Human Dimensions of Change*. Crown Copyright April 2005, Department of Health Publications, London. www.library.nhs.uk/knowledgemanagement/ViewResource.aspx?resID=156458.

Improvement Leaders Guides (2005b) Gateway reference 4701. *Process Mapping, Analysis and Redesign*. Crown Copyright April 2005, Department of Health Publications, PO Box 77, London. www.library.nhs.uk/healthmanagement/ViewResource.aspx?resID=70171.

Oshry, B. (1996) *Seeing Systems: Unlocking the Mysteries of Organisational Life*, paperback edn. Berret-Koehler Publishers, San Francisco.

Raelin, J.A. (2003) *Creating Leaderful Organisations: How to Bring Out the Leadership in Everyone*. Berrett-Koehler Publishers, San Francisco.

Reeves, T. (1998) *Alchemy for Managers: Turning Experience into Achievement*, revised edn. Butterworth-Heinemann, Oxford.

Revans, R. (1998) *ABC of Action Learning: Empowering Managers to Act and to Learn from Action*. Lemos and Crane, London.

Senge, P.M. (1990) *The Fifth Discipline: The Art and Practice of the Learning Organisation*. Random House, London.

Visser, C. and Bodien, G.S. (no date). *Solution-Focused Coaching: Simply Effective*. www.thesolutionfocus.com/effective.doc 24.01.06.

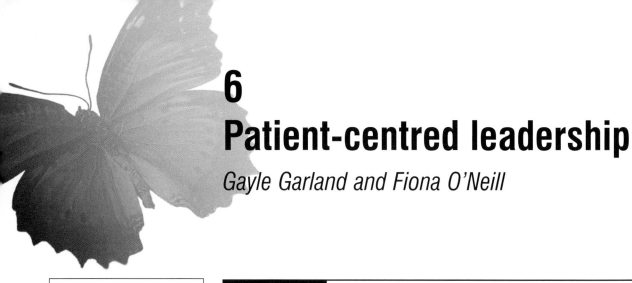

6
Patient-centred leadership
Gayle Garland and Fiona O'Neill

○━ Keywords
....

Patient-centred leadership

Is expressly intended to provide a good service and a positive emotional experience for each patient, as defined by that patient

Introduction

In this chapter we explore **patient-centred leadership**, that is, the leadership of health care and services designed around the needs of patients. More than any other type of leadership described in this book, patient-centred leadership is a shared responsibility. No one person or organisation can achieve patient-centred health services, it takes the combined experience and perspectives of many people, each one holding a valuable piece of the puzzle.

Everyone involved – patients and their family members, health professionals, managers and staff – agrees that high-quality, patient-centred care and service is what we all expect and deserve. The challenge is that patient-centred care means different things to different people.

Reflective activity

Imagine that you are waiting in the A&E department with your child who has had a fever and has been vomiting for the past 24 hours. You notice a sign that says, 'Ward Philosophy – We are committed to providing high-quality, patient-centred care at all times'.

● What would that mean to you? What would you expect from the staff?

● If you were a staff nurse on that ward, what would the sign mean to you? How would the ward managers expect the staff to meet the commitment stated in the ward philosophy?

● If you were the chief executive of the trust, how would you define high-quality, patient-centred care for the child with the fever, and what would you want to see the health professionals in A&E doing?

We will look in more depth at the various meanings of 'patient-centred care' later in this chapter, but we will first explore the origins and evolution of patient-centred care.

The road from profession-centred to patient-centred health care

The National Health Service (NHS) has come a long way from its inception in 1948. Not only have there been monumental changes in medical treatment and professional practice, there have also been fundamental changes in the relationship between the government, the NHS, health professionals and the public. Because the NHS is large and complex, changes are not always easy or quick.

Profession-centred health care

> In the case of nutrition and health, just as in the case of education, the Gentlemen of Whitehall really do know better what is good for the people than the people know themselves.
>
> Jay (1937)

This quote is from a civil servant named Douglas Jay, and it captures the thinking that shaped the formation of the NHS in 1948. Since the nineteenth century, those who could not afford to pay for health care had received treatment provided by charitable organisations or through a network of services for the poor funded by the local authority. By quite early in the twentieth century, the demand for care was too great for the charities and local authorities to manage. It was recognised that for the country to rebuild following two world wars, a fit and healthy population would be needed. The patchwork of health services that existed prior to the formation of the NHS was simply not up to the job.

The NHS was also part of a civilised society built on socialist ideals, two of which were built into the design of the NHS. The first ideal is that everyone should have equal access to health care services, regardless of their ability to pay or the nature of their need. The NHS was therefore set up to be free at the point of delivery and available to all citizens from 'cradle to grave'. The second socialist ideal built into the initial design of the NHS was that the better off in society (the wealthy, business owners and middle-class professionals) were expected to help the less well off. The way to accomplish this was to pay for the NHS out of general taxation, because those who were better off financially paid more taxes. Poor people paid the least in taxes and yet were entitled to the same health services as the wealthy (Timmins, 1995).

In the early days of the NHS, the general public had virtually no say about health services or even their own health care. The advice of health professionals, particularly doctors, was followed without question. When it came to designing health services for the public, doctors were also seen as the experts.

The NHS was the result of many hours of discussion and compromise between government ministers and a range of organisations and professional interest groups. The medical profession took centre stage in the often fierce negotiations. Many doctors were fearful that the government would interfere with the practice of medicine, and with the doctor's right to make decisions about treatment. An understanding between doctors and the government was eventually reached that cleared the way for the formation of the NHS. The understanding was that doctors would retain autonomy over their work, and, in return, doctors accepted that the government had control over the purse strings.

In 1948, the health care system was **paternalistic**. Paternalism often creates dependency and encourages people to sit back and let others decide what is best for them. Doctors and nurses were the holders of unique information to which the public had no access, and so a culture of 'doctor/nurse knows best' became the norm, with doctors and nurses making decisions on behalf of patients without active involvement from patients and carers. In general, doctors and nurses enjoyed a high degree of respect and were treated with deference and compliance by patients and government officials. It was health professionals that determined the way that health services were designed. It was accepted that the public would take no part in determining standards and priorities, or have any real influence over the type of services provided. It was to be many years before concepts like choice, quality and shared decision making were to enter the picture. Patients were cast in a passive role as the grateful, uncomplaining recipients of the 'gift' of state-funded health care in a system characterised by the almost unbridled power of the professions. The patient's role was just that – to be patient and to accept stoically and without question the wisdom of professional experts and the shortfalls of the system.

Patient-centred health care begins

The public confidence in the government's ability to run the NHS came into question in the 1960s. Some would argue that it was no surprise that standards were poor in the NHS, considering that the health service had to compete with other public services for funds and that, in post-war Britain, there was never enough money to go around. A series of inquiries and reports was published that highlighted very poor standards of care and inhumane conditions in the large institutions and geriatric wards that were home to increasing numbers of elderly and mentally ill people. *Sans Everything: A Case to Answer* (Barton, 1967), for example, was a moving and disturbing account of the neglect, indifference and boredom that marked the daily life of many elderly patients on geriatric wards. This and, among others, the official inquiry into conditions at Ely Hospital, an institution for people with learning disabilities, led to moves to strengthen government control over standards.

The reports also influenced the creation of pressure groups representing patients' interests, such as the Patients Association and AEGIS (Aid to the Elderly in Government Institutions). Community Health Councils were introduced in 1974 and were the first attempt to formally represent the public's interest in the NHS.

○━π *Keywords*

Paternalistic
Describes a system where actions, decisions, rules or policies that relate to patients' 'best interests' are taken without considering the patient's own beliefs, preferences, value systems and knowledge

This growing concern about standards in the NHS, especially in relation to the provision of services for older people, people with mental illness and people with chronic health problems, came at the same time as the start of a more general economic downturn. Steep rises in oil prices plunged the global economy into a recession, and unemployment began to rise. Money was even tighter than before, but the public clearly wanted health services to receive attention. When Mrs Thatcher was elected in 1979, the government committed to a programme of radical reform of the NHS.

From patients to consumers

In 1983, Sir Roy Griffiths, Chief Executive of the Sainsbury supermarket group, was asked by Mrs Thatcher to conduct a management review of the NHS. The review showed that the health service was inefficient, devoid of effective scrutiny, and largely self-serving.

> Businessmen have a keen sense of how well they are looking after their customers. Whether the NHS is meeting the needs of the patient and the community, and can prove that it is doing so, is open to question.
>
> Klein (2001, p. 128)

In an effort to address the failings of the system, it was decided to introduce a system of general management into the NHS. Prior to this, the NHS had been run mostly by health professionals, doctors and nurses in particular. Health professionals generally had no formal education in management, and there was a belief that professional managers would bring 'value for money' into the health service and create more 'customer satisfaction', as was the case in business. This meant that managers who were not clinical people had responsibility for looking at costs and outcomes of treatment. This signalled the end of the 'understanding' between professional groups and the government that had survived largely intact since 1948. Professions no longer had complete autonomy over clinical practice; they were challenged by managers to consider cost, patient satisfaction and clinical outcomes. Clinical professionals became accountable for the first time to people outside their professional group, though it would be many years before clinical practices were challenged in any meaningful way.

Another important result of the Griffiths report (1983) was for the government to begin to think of the public as consumers of health care services rather than the recipients of public charity. The choice of the word 'consumer' was an important step towards patient-centred services, because consumers had rights under the law. The *Patient's Charter* (Department of Health, 1996) set out for the first time the rights and standards that patients could expect from the health service. The standards were not particularly ambitious. Klein (2001) argues that the standards really did highlight how professionally dominated the NHS had become. For example, the Charter gave the right to 'be guaranteed admission for a treatment by a specific date no later than 2 years from the day when your consultant places you on a waiting list'. Another standard was that outpatients are given a specific appointment time and will be seen within 30 minutes of that time. That standard was meant to stop the common practice of block booking of outpatient clinics that may have suited the professional staff, but took no account of the waiting time that had to be stoically endured by patients. It is interesting to note that the original patient's charter, only 10-years-old, is no longer available from the Department of Health: an indication, perhaps, of just how far the standards for patient-centred care have moved on.

Although members of the public were officially classified as consumers and were accorded some rights under the law, in reality the public still had very little 'consumer power'. One of the primary sources of consumer power is choice. For example, if I stay in a hotel that has dirty rooms or poor service, I will choose to stay somewhere else in the future. If enough people make the same choice that I did, then the hotel will either improve, so that it regains the trust of the customer, or go out of business. However, because there is only one NHS, there is no real option to 'take your business elsewhere'.

If you were dissatisfied with the services of the NHS, there was nowhere else to go. The most powerful tool of the consumer – choice – did not yet exist. Unless patients were willing to seek treatment outside the NHS, and to pay for it, the situation was still very much 'take it or leave it'.

From consumers to partners

The Griffiths report (1983) was not the only lever for change in the 1980s and 1990s. The country was undergoing a period of rapid social, economic and technological change. The UK was becoming an increasingly wealthy society and people's expectations for their own health and quality of life were rising, as were their expectations about health services and the people who deliver them. The Internet has given the public access to information on health conditions that was previously only available to professionals.

By the 1990s, the trust in and respect for doctors and nurses that were common in the early days of the NHS were no longer guaranteed. There was a series of high-profile failures, incompetence and deceptions by health professionals that changed the relationship between them and the public forever. In 1991, Beverley Allitt, a newly qualified nurse in a children' hospital, was convicted of killing four children and injuring nine others. The inquiry into the case found that colleagues working alongside Allitt were alarmed by the increase in child deaths and near deaths, but because they could not believe that someone would deliberately harm patients under their care, Allitt's crime spree continued (Allitt Inquiry, 1991). The public blamed the doctors, the nurses and the managers for the deaths. A shadow was cast over the whole idea of 'professional self-regulation' – after all, the doctors and nurses seemed incapable of identifying and stopping a rogue nurse. The public also blamed the hospital management for failing to put into place a system that would have spotted these abnormalities sooner.

Since then, two other cases in particular have raised questions about the effectiveness of professionals and managers to protect the public from harm at the hands of health professionals. The inquiry into excessive death rates for the children's heart surgery team at Bristol Royal Infirmary (Department of Health, 2001a) revealed that a consultant anaesthetist raised concerns with other doctors, including the chief executive of the trust who was a doctor, and yet no effective action was taken. The anaesthetist was ostracised by his colleagues as a 'whistle blower' and left the country to practise medicine abroad. Many months went by, during which time more children died, until effective comparisons were made between Bristol and other heart centres that showed the inadequacy of the care.

The public inquiry into the children's heart surgery team at Bristol Royal Infirmary, and the subsequent report known as the Kennedy Report, highlighted the devastating impact of poor organisation, ineffective teamworking, lack of leadership, paternalism and a system that did not put patients at the centre of care. A number of children died while under the care of the Bristol team, and it took a long time for the comparative differences in mortality rates at Bristol to be effectively investigated. The report calls for a culture of openness and honesty, and makes specific recommendations about the need for patients to be involved in decision making. The report also includes a strong focus on the information needs of patients, not only about their own treatment options but also about the standards of care available to them and other non-clinical aspects of patients' experience.

✍ *Over to you*

In *Learning from Bristol: The Report of the Public Inquiry into Children's Heart Surgery at the Bristol Royal Infirmary 1984–1995* (Bristol Royal Infirmary Inquiry, 2001), the government addressed all the recommendations and called for a new relationship between the government and the NHS and the NHS and patients, recognising the need for fundamental reform in order to deliver 'high-quality, patient-centred services' where patients are enabled to 'become equal partners with health care professionals'.

Access the final report via www.bristol-inquiry.org.uk/final_report/index.htm.

Aim to read at least the summary and recommendations and consider how you could usefully apply the learning to your own experience and working environment.

The Over to you feature highlights the fact that patient involvement in all aspects of their care and the design of services is not just a 'nicety': it is a necessity for safe, satisfying and effective care.

In the second case, the inquiry into the murders committed by GP Harold Shipman found that the GPs, nurses and receptionists working alongside Shipman were unaware of the high number of deaths among his patients. Shipman's friendly, easy-going manner and his reputation as a 'nice man and a good doctor' caused patients and colleagues to support him, even when he was under police investigation. In the end, the alarm was raised by family members of the patients whom he had killed. It seemed in this case, and many others, that neither management systems nor health professionals could be counted on to identify and act on dangerous or inadequate practice (Shipman Inquiry, 2004).

What exactly is patient-centred care?

In the activity at the beginning of this chapter, I asked you to think about how you would define 'patient-centred care' from the point of view of the patient, family, staff nurse, manager, and chief executive. The chances are that there were some common themes that emerged from your reflection.

In the role of a patient or family member, you probably wanted the child to be seen quickly and receive safe and effective care; to be kept informed, and to be given options where possible. As a staff nurse, you may have defined patient-centred care in much the same way, and yet you will be challenged to provide patient-centred care to all the patients presenting at A&E. This may mean that some patients have to wait whilst those with more severe conditions are treated. The mother of the child who has to wait may not believe that the child is getting patient-centred care.

As a manager, you would want to ensure that all the standards for admission and treatment times are met as well as that individual patients receive personalised care. Meeting these targets not only ensures that all patients receive a baseline standard of service but also that the trust receives the recognition and funding that goes with the attainment of targets.

As chief executive, you may want to ensure that services are provided to the standards expected, within budget, and that the public and the community are satisfied with their care. You would want to ensure that patients are represented on trust committees and that their concerns are addressed.

A study by the Kings Fund (Corben and Rosen, 2005) found that various professional groups already see themselves as offering patient-centred care. Those professional groups also had diverse definitions of patient-centred care. Whilst this finding is encouraging, it is also a concern. The danger is that, when health professionals believe that they already offer patient-centred services, they may not be using the same yardstick as the patients. For example, members of a GP practice may see themselves as patient centred because every weekday they hold open clinics without the need for appointments. Whilst this is welcomed by many patients, it may not be what is most needed. In neighbourhoods where many people commute to work, patients may want GP appointments to be available in the evening or at weekends; for them, open clinics on weekdays are still not convenient.

Hospitals may also fall short of being patient centred in the eyes of the patient. Whilst the quality of food in hospital has risen in recent years, it is still common for there to be little food available after 6.00 p.m., and what is available is usually cold. This could result in a patient's being admitted from A&E in the evening and having no access to food for a long period. Health professionals see themselves as providing patient-centred care because the quality and choice of food has improved, but the patients' need for food in the evening remains unmet.

Another hurdle to overcome along the road to patient-centred care is that patients are used to fitting in around health services and may not even consider asking for something else. Whilst the public expects private hospitals to be modern, clean and nicely decorated, they expect much less from their local NHS hospital. Paradoxically, even though the public's expectations for the NHS have risen, these expectations may still be less than the public deserves.

Reflective activity

Think about what changes to the health service you would ask for if anything were possible? Would it be airline-style, online appointment booking? Would it be a mobile service that comes to your door? Perhaps it would be aromatherapy sessions on weekday evenings. What would you want?

What the research says

There is a growing body of evidence that can help us to understand what is important from a patient and public perspective. Based on extensive survey data, the Picker Institute (2005) has identified eight aspects of health care that patients consider most important:

- fast access to reliable health care
- effective treatment delivered by trusted professionals
- involvement in decisions and respect for preferences
- clear, comprehensive information and support for self-care
- attention to physical and environmental needs
- emotional support, empathy and respect

- involvement of, and support for, family and carers
- continuity of care and smooth transitions.

Reflective activity

Think about how well this list reflects your expectations of the health service. What is most important to you? What would you add?

The National Consumer Council (2004) asked members of the public to identify the public service 'X' factor that differentiates the best providers from the run-of-the-mill providers. People most often mentioned values that relate to the human aspects of service provision, including empathy, compassion, respect, and taking the time to listen and respond to individual circumstances. Research conducted as part of the national consultation for the strategy paper *Building on the Best: Choice, Responsiveness and Equity in the NHS* (Department of Health, 2003) also demonstrated the importance of addressing the emotional experience of patients and found that many people felt that the NHS was not particularly good at meeting emotional needs.

People involved in the research shared the same opinion about what a positive patient experience at an emotional level should feel like. Patients want to feel reassured, confident, cared for, informed, safe and relaxed. Of particular importance was feeling that they are important and 'special'. Several positive feelings that people wanted to have during their journey, as well as the feelings that people would like to have as a result of their experience, were identified (Department of Health, 2005a).

The meaning of patient-centred care is becoming clearer as a result of these studies and the experience of professionals and managers working

Table 6.1 Feelings related to patient journey and experience

Feelings during the patient journey	Feelings resulting from patient experience
Reassured	Satisfied
Respected	Relieved
Cared for	Cared for
Listened to	Confident in treatment and the NHS as a whole
In control	Pride
Safe	

with patients and the public. It is important to remember, however, that the expectations of patients and public will continue to evolve as will the definition of patient-centred care. Whilst the characteristics listed in the table provide a guide to standards of service and care, individuals differ, and it is wise to check with each patient to ensure that their needs are met.

Patient-centred leadership

It is clear from research reports that patients want both a good service and a good emotional experience. In patient-centred leadership, the leader's actions will differ depending on their role and on the relationship with the patient.

The role of government in patient-centred leadership

The main role of the government is to turn the public's values into public policy. One of the main challenges to any government is to determine public values and to align public policy with those values. Whilst not all members of the public want the same thing, there are definitely trends in public opinion. For example, research conducted more than 20 years ago showed that smoking was harmful. If public policy was driven by research, smoking would have been banned years ago. Public policy is much more closely aligned with public opinion, and 20 years ago the public was not willing for the government to take any action against smoking. Little by little, health policy has shifted to reflect the public's change of mood on smoking. One of the first actions taken by the policy makers was to restrict the sale of tobacco, so that it should not be sold to people under a certain age. Then warning labels were required on cigarette packets. Smoking in government buildings and hospitals was finally banned, and, from 2007, there will be a ban on smoking in public places. There comes a tipping point where public values shift, and the public expects policy to reflect those values.

The public values for the health service are very different today from when the health service started. The New Labour Government that came to power in 1997 made modernising the health service a key priority because that is what the public was demanding. The White Paper *Modernising Government* (Cabinet Office, 1999) outlined the themes of responsiveness, innovation, and improvement that were to drive the programme of 'renewal and reform' of public services. The document made reference to ensuring that service providers could meet the needs of a public 'accustomed to consumer choice and consumption in the private sector'.

Professional groups and individuals were asked for their views on health service reforms, but, more than ever before, the views of the public were sought and considered. Policy makers have a number of ways to find out the public's views. It is quite common now for the government to undertake a consultation on health policy changes before finalising them. Draft policies are posted on the Department of Health website and members of the public are invited to comment. National and local surveys or focus groups are held to discuss some issues. Of course, the government also depends on the public to write, phone, text and email their views to their local Members of Parliament. Groups that represent patients are often asked for their views. Age Concern is consulted about policies that would affect older people, and MIND helps the government to relate to the issues of people with mental illness. The views of the public carry more weight today than ever before.

The role of the government is not limited to implementing public values of the moment. Leading patient-centred services is also about planning for the future by anticipating changes in society and technology that will affect health services. The population of the UK is aging, and we are seeing a shift from acute to chronic health problems as people live longer. The rapid increase in numbers of people living with long-term health conditions is a poor match for a system geared to providing care for patients with short-term, self-contained illness (WHO, 2005). This trend requires health services to change, and the people with those conditions are important in leading those changes.

National service frameworks (NSF) are one of the ways that the government leads service development. Most NSFs deal with long-term conditions such as cancer, heart disease, mental illness, and diabetes, which are increasingly common in the UK. NSFs set standards for not only the clinical treatment of these conditions but also for service standards such as speed of treatment. The NSF for cancer, for example, states that a patient must be seen by a cancer specialist within a very short time of diagnosis.

Probably the most important policies that lead us towards a more patient-centred health service are those that set general standards about how health services are delivered. In particular, targets have been set for waiting times for appointments, consultations, surgery and emergency treatment. The original promises set out in the Patient's Charter are being brought into line with modern service standards. For example, the waiting times for surgery were originally set at two years in the Patient's Charter, and now trusts are required to admit patients within six months of their being placed on a waiting list. The waiting times are set to be reduced even further: to 18 weeks by the end of 2008 (Department of Health, 2004).

The NHS Plan (Department of Health, 2000) included a chapter on patient involvement and outlined a number of new roles and structures. The Patient Advocacy and Liaison Service (PALS) was created to provide an independent source of advice and support for patients. There was also a requirement for all NHS trusts to establish Patients' Forums and to make their board meetings open to the public. Following on in that vein, the Health and Social Care Act 2001 requires all NHS institutions to make arrangements to involve and consult patients and the public.

Through consulting with the public and enacting policies that reflect the public's expectations, the government becomes the voice of the people in leading health services. Health policy is becoming more patient centred by requiring trusts and professionals to meet clinical and service standards. Public policy also requires professionals and organisations to make information more widely available, and to demonstrate consideration and involvement of patients and the public at all levels.

Evidence base

We recommend that you read:

Department of Health (2000) *The NHS Plan: A Plan for Investment, a Plan for Reform*, The Stationery Office, London. Chapter 10, Changes for Patients, pp. 88–95.
National Consumer Council (2004) *Making Public Services Personal: A New Compact for Public Services*. NCC: London. Executive Summary, pp. 7–12.

Patient-centred leadership in health care provider organisations

Patient-centred leadership in health care provider organisations involves making it possible for staff to care both *for* and *about* patients. These leadership priorities are two sides of the same coin. Patients expect that service standards such as waiting times will be honoured, and that services will be coordinated and convenient. Patients also expect that staff will be pleasant and knowledgeable and will assist them as needed.

Leaders in health care provider organisations have different roles. Senior managers, executives and directors are primarily responsible for ensuring that service standards are met, whilst front-line managers are responsible for ensuring that staff members deliver a good experience for the patient. Both types of leadership are needed; if the staff members do not have the drugs and supplies to treat patients then it is unlikely that they can deliver a good experience.

Patient-centred leadership by front-line managers and leaders

Front-line managers are the people who are responsible for running a department on a daily basis. The relationship between the front-line manager and those people delivering care is one of the most important factors in staff satisfaction and team effectiveness (Aston University, 1999). How staff members feel about their roles and the relationships at work will often determine how they behave towards the patients. Those who feel respected and empowered by their managers will usually extend respect and empowerment to their patients.

The first task of a patient-centred leader at the front line is therefore to be relentlessly focused on the human experience of staff and patients. Kotter and Cohen (2002) argue that successful leadership of organisations is about changing the *behaviour* of people. Most often people will be persuaded to change their behaviour because they *feel* that it is the right thing to do. Kotter and Cohen summarise their argument as follows:

> Our main finding, put simply, is that the central issue is never strategy, culture or systems. All those elements and others are important. But the core of the matter is always about changing the behaviour of people, and behaviour change happens in highly successful situations mostly by speaking to people's feelings.
>
> Kotter and Cohen (2002, p. x)

Whilst staff members may not be persuaded to change long-established practices because of a new policy document or a new directive from the government or trust board, their close association with the experiences of the patients can create a compelling reason to change. For example, despite every health professional understanding the importance of hand washing in infection control and prevention, studies show that the rates of actual hand washing can be very low. Health professionals do not intend to circumvent the rules: it is time consuming to wash hands between every patient contact, and busy people simply do not have enough time. Making hand hygiene more convenient by providing alcohol gel at every bedside is one way that managers can demonstrate their understanding and respect for the experience of staff and that they are working to make the work lives of staff more satisfying.

Failing to pay attention to the experience of staff members can result in their failing to pay attention to the experience of the patient.

Reflective activity

'I said to the nurse, please feed her'

This was the headline of an article in *The Guardian* newspaper (7 January 2006) written by the author Blake Morrison. Morrison outlines a number of cases, including that of his mother-in-law, of elderly people receiving inadequate care in British hospitals. The article describes how new pressure groups, for example Patient Protect, are starting; such groups lobby for better standards and give advice to worried relatives who are concerned about how to ensure that their loved ones get what they need in hospital.

You may be aware of other recent articles in the press and on TV.

- What do you think about when you read or hear something about less-than-adequate care for people in the NHS?
- Is such care related to poor leadership at the front line?
- What can you as a leader do to ensure that poor care does not happen?

Patient-centred leadership by senior managers

Senior managers are responsible for ensuring that service standards and targets are met and that funds are managed effectively. Because health care provider organisations are better managed and better financed than ever before, waiting times have dropped and services have improved remarkably in the past few years. Unfortunately, sometimes senior managers' focus on targets and finances can cause front-line managers and staff to lose sight of the patient experience.

In order to stay patient focused, senior managers need to listen to front-line managers and staff. The following patient-centred leadership actions for senior managers have been recommended by participants in national programmes for front-line leadership offered between 2000 and 2005.

- Front-line staff members judge the culture of the organisation by the behaviour of their front-line managers. Most front-line staff want to improve the patient experience but are powerless without the support of their managers. Seeing their managers being called upon to deal with service issues and targets, staff can start to believe that meeting targets is the only thing that matters. Senior managers need therefore to be sure that they communicate the importance of achieving a positive patient experience; paying attention to only one of these factors is not enough.

- Front-line staff and managers need to see that senior managers are there for the patients' benefit and not just to manage the budget. Performance updates should take a back seat in communications with front-line staff, as that will send a message that being patient centred is most important

  (Garland, 2006)

Here is a good example of a senior manager demonstrating patient-centred leadership.

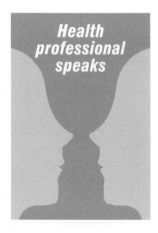

Health professional speaks

Ward housekeeper

The 'mother test'

Our chief executive is very patient focused. He personally comes to every induction programme for new staff and speaks about mental illness and the type of difficulties that bring people to our hospital. He says that we should treat every individual here as we ourselves would like to be treated or how we would wish our mothers to be treated should they find themselves needing care. I always remember that: respect is everything.

The role of development

So far, we have discussed two important strategies for patient-centred leadership in provider organisations. The first strategy is for front-line managers to pay particular attention to the experience of patients and staff, and to work to make that experience more satisfying. This is achieved by treating the staff with respect, valuing their contribution and involving them in decision making. This in turn encourages staff to honour the values and beliefs of the patients and, therefore, to deliver patient-centred care.

The second strategy is for senior managers to ensure the effective running of the organisation, but not at the expense of patient experience. A senior manager who communicates the importance of meeting targets from the patient's point of view will have a greater chance of influencing staff.

Another strategy for patient-centred leadership is to make staff development available. Staff development is one way of showing staff that they are valued, but staff development also has a patient-centred purpose. In particular, staff development programmes that require staff to apply their learning have a direct benefit to the patient as well as reinforcing a patient-centred culture. Leadership at the Point of Care is a national programme for front-line staff that has many examples of how staff members make small changes that improve care (Henley Management College, 2005). Staff return from the programme with a new sense of connection with the patient experience and are eager to implement their ideas; in organisations where they receive support from their peers and managers, the programme has been successful in improving care.

Also directly beneficial to patient care is the systematic practice development programme whereby, through a framework of standards and an active coaching process, teams set out to improve care as they learn. Encouraging this form of team and personal development is a way for organisations to be patient centred.

The role of health professionals in patient-centred leadership

Health care professionals demonstrate patient-centred leadership by considering and accommodating the values, preferences and needs of individual patients in their professional interactions, and by applying what has been learnt from close patient contact to inform strategic planning and service development. Because patients expect both a good service and a good experience, it is important for the professional to try to meet both needs.

Faced with increasing demands and a rapidly changing service, stretched practitioners can fall into the trap of seeing patients as a burden rather than a resource. If patients are to be actively involved in health care, there needs to be a new dimension to the relationship between patients and professionals, so that the expertise and knowledge of patients and the wider community can be harnessed for the benefit of all. Whilst some patients, through the severity of their illness or personal choice, may not wish to be actively involved in decision making or in contributing to service development, there is plenty of evidence that indicates that service users' desire and capacity for involvement in decision making is higher than professionals often acknowledge (Coulter, 2002).

In three 'messages', Harry Cayton (2005) neatly summarises why patient and public involvement should be seen as a given rather than an optional extra in today's NHS:

- **Trust me I'm a patient**. I use the services you provide. I have views on how you could make them better for me and the people in my community. I understand my illness better than you do – I am the one suffering from it. I have views to offer about the way I am treated. Trust me; listen to me; trust my expertise – we can both benefit from this relationship.

- **Tell me the truth**. I know that the NHS has a strong political influence. I know that there are uncertainties in medical practice. But I have the right to be given the opportunity to understand what these are, to make choices about my care, to be involved in the service I pay for. Share the truth with me.

- **Nothing about us without us**. You decide on our behalf the services you think we want, and how you think we want them. Ask us; involve us in your decisions. Bring us inside for the benefit of all (Cayton, 2005).

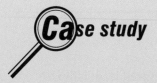

Case study

Two approaches to meeting patient needs

Approach A

Surgeon A is a young woman, full of energy and efficiency. During Mrs Z's appointment, she tells Mrs Z that surgery is needed and that she is scheduling her at the end of the month on a Wednesday. Mrs Z is told to come with a bag and be ready to stay five days. She starts to tell the surgeon that she has a problem with child care that week, but the surgeon interrupts her to say that she is the best surgeon for this type of problem and that she is very busy. She warns that if Mrs Z does not take that surgery time, she will go to the bottom of the list and will not get her surgery for months. The surgeon tells Mrs Z to call her office with her decision tomorrow and leaves the room.

Approach B

Surgeon B is a middle-aged man, with half glasses and a bow tie. He sits down with Mrs Z and discusses the type of surgery that he recommends, including the risks and benefits. He explains that there is an opening at the end of the month for the surgery. When Mrs Z explains that she would not be able to attend then because of difficulties with child care, Surgeon B gives her the phone number of the booking service and encourages her to call and see what she can work out with them. He goes on to explain that she may have to wait up to six months for the surgery, but he does not believe that the wait will make the condition worse. Surgeon B adds that he will write to her GP, explaining ways that the latter can help her manage her condition during the wait if need be. He makes it clear that he is willing to look again at her needs if the situation changes.

- Which interaction is more patient centred?
- How do you think the patient will feel following Surgeon B's approach?

Surgeon A behaves in a profession-centred way. She gives the patient a 'take it or leave it' choice, and shows no sensitivity to the emotional experience of the patient. It is likely that the patient will be upset by the situation and feel less confident in the surgeon.

Surgeon B shows a more patient-centred approach. When the patient is not able to take the surgery date at the end of the month, he gives her information to help her manage the wait, and to reassure her. He may not be able to arrange for her surgery date to be moved up, but he has done his best to assist her to manage the situation.

Empathy

Empathy is an important facet of patient-centred leadership. Empathy allows you to concentrate on the other person and incorporates notions of respect and effective communication. Empathy is both an emotional quality and behavioural. When interacting with patients, you need to demonstrate active, empathetic listening. Empathetic listening means listening not only for the facts, but also for the emotional impact of the situation. Facts and emotions together create a rich picture of the patient experience as a whole. A rich picture is a very useful tool for exercising patient-centred leadership. Let me illustrate.

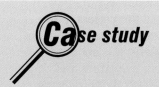
Case study

Protected meal times or early assessment?

Sandra is convinced that protected meal times should be introduced on the ward. The therapists with whom she works are reluctant to agree since it would require them to change the workflow in their department, potentially causing a delay in initial assessments. It is important that the initial assessments for therapy happen early in the course of treatment, as delays cause the patients to become weaker and less

continued

mobile. The therapists regard the early assessment of the patient as patient-centred care, and they are reluctant to see the standard slip. Sandra is invited to attend their staff meeting and needs to decide her approach. She considers three possibilities.

1. Prepare a detailed chart of the following data: therapy appointments within an hour of meal time, the number of times a patient's meal is interrupted, the number of patients at risk nutritionally, and their weights and percentage meal consumption. Sandra's hope is that the therapists will be persuaded by the data and be convinced of the benefits of her idea.

2. Sandra has been noting whenever a patient has an interruption to their meal time for therapy. She has been asking each person what they think of having their meal interrupted for therapy. Most patients are unhappy about their meals being interrupted, and, with a little prompting from her, they have provided some comments. She has recorded all their statements but is only planning to share the 'unhappy' statements with the therapy staff. Sandra is hoping that the therapy staff will realise how unhappy the patients are and that they will be persuaded to change.

3. Sandra collects some numerical data plus the patient's experiences (good and bad) and shares both at the meeting. She is hoping to have a discussion that comes up with a solution that will be in the patients' best interests.

Which strategy do you think will be most effective and why?

The first option is an example of relaying fact without impact. Facts without context and meaning can sound hollow and pedantic. It is not unusual to get a shrug of the shoulders and a 'so what?' response to a lot of data. The human impact is missing and there is no compelling reason to change the way that things are done.

The second option is an example of playing to emotions that have a tenuous attachment to fact. It is almost as if the staff member is setting out to collect complaints in an effort to force the therapy staff to change. This is not an example of being patient centred. It is in fact a form of paternalism where patients are manipulated with the intention of achieving the aims of the staff member.

The third option represents the most balanced and honest approach. It is an attempt to convey a rich picture of experiences from patients who have had interruptions to their meal times. Subjective and objective information is presented; good and bad experiences are portrayed. This approach is more likely to engender cooperation from the therapists and represents the most patient-centred approach of all.

Patient-centred leadership from health professionals is evident in the nature of interactions between the professional and the patient, and among professionals about the patient. Patient-centred leadership is not about blind compliance with every wish of the patient. It is about seeking, acknowledging and adapting care to reflect the values and preferences of the patients wherever possible. It is also about applying what you learnt from practising patient-centred leadership in such a way as to improve the patient focus of future care.

The role of patients and carers in patient-centred leadership

It may seem obvious, but the role of the patient in leading patient-centred care is to communicate with health professionals, managers and others in such a way as to make their preference, values, needs and expectations known. Further, it is to relay not only the facts, but the experience of being a patient in such a way as to influence managers and professionals for the benefit of other patients.

This responsibility may be difficult to fulfil. It is common for the patient to feel that the health professional is more knowledgeable and experienced than they are. Patients have to rely on health professionals to meet their needs, and they can feel reluctant to challenge. When interacting with patients and carers, it is best to assume that they will feel at a disadvantage around health professionals. Feeling at a disadvantage can result in a number of responses:

- **Lack of confidence and an unwillingness to speak up**. This is perhaps the most common patient response. Rather than express their needs or preferences, they 'suffer in silence', never giving the professional the chance to meet their needs. This is a recipe for dissatisfaction on both sides of the relationship.

- **Anger**. Unmet needs can build a frustration and resentment that can end in unpleasantness. Helping the patient to express their needs and state their expectations will usually prevent the worst outbreaks.

- **Complaints**. It is not uncommon for a patient to wait until after their treatment is over to express their discontent. This is unfortunate in that it is often too late then to repair the damage, and, again, both parties end up dissatisfied.

(Dickson, 2004)

The key to patients taking their proper place in the leadership of patient-centred care is not only in enabling patients to feel confident in sharing their views with others but also in enabling them to participate effectively in a setting in which they may feel a lack of confidence.

The next chapter will explore strategies for achieving effective involvement; for now, let us consider the future of patient-centred leadership.

Beyond patient-centred to patient-led

In 2005, the idea that the NHS should not be only be patient centred but patient led took centre stage. *Creating a Patient-led NHS* outlines how the NHS needs to move on from 'being an organisation which simply delivers services to people to being one which is totally patient led, responding to their needs and wishes' (Department of Health, 2005b).

Evidence base

Read Department of Health (2005b) *Creating a Patient-led NHS: Delivering the NHS Improvement Plan*. Department of Health, London.

Every aspect of the new system is designed to create a service which is patient led, where:

- People have a far greater range of choices and of information and help to make choices.
- There are stronger standards and safeguards for patients.
- NHS organisations are better at understanding patients and their needs, use new and different methodologies to do so and have better and more regular sources of information about preferences and satisfaction.

(Department of Health, 2005b)

Patient-led service is about more than service development and choice. In 2001, the Chief Medical Officer outlined a new approach to patient involvement in the management of their chronic diseases. The 'Expert Patient' programme aims to 'empower and liberate patients to play a central role in decisions about their illness' (Department of Health, 2001b). The programme is now embedded into the NHS, and the expectation is that anyone who has a long-term illness will be able to access a programme in their local area. Facilitated by people who have a long-term condition and based on principles of self-management, the programme aims to decrease dependency on the health care system and promote independence and empowerment.

Reflective activity

Imagine a truly patient-led NHS.

Think about and describe the type of services available. What are the health professionals doing? How are services paid for? Are people healthier? Are patients happier?

Reflective activity

A family has just moved into your area. They have a child with physical and mental disability as a result of a head injury suffered when the child was three years old. The child is now seven, and the mother is pregnant with her second child. How would you interact with this family to plan for their needs:

- using a profession-centred approach?
- using a patient-centred approach?
- using a patient-led approach?

Reflective activity

- Describe a time when you demonstrated patient-centred leadership.
- How else can you demonstrate patient-centred leadership?

Summary

In this chapter, we have taken a journey through the NHS from its beginnings as a paternalistic, profession-centred organisation and on into its future as a patient-led service. We have explored the meaning of patient-centred care from a variety of perspectives and have discussed some of the challenges faced by health care professionals, their organisations and the patients themselves.

Patient-centred leadership is simply leading in a patient-centred way. Acting in a patient-centred way means that the values, beliefs and preferences of the patient are sought, respected, and incorporated into services wherever possible. Whether you are a chief executive, a manager, a health care professional, or a patient, you have a role in patient-centred leadership. It will take the commitment and participation of many people to realise the vision of a patient-led NHS.

> ### ℞℞℞℞℞**Rapid recap**
>
> Check your progress so far by working through each of the following questions:
>
> 1. Provide a working definition of the term 'patient-centred care'.
> 2. Identify at least four important events or changes that have occurred since the beginnings of the NHS that have contributed to current reforms.
> 3. What is the main role of the government in patient-led services?
> 4. Describe at least one action that health care provider organisations or senior managers can take to move services toward patient-centred provision.
> 5. Define 'empathy' and its role in patient-centred leadership.
> 6. What is meant by the term a 'patient-led NHS'?
>
> If you have difficulty with more than one of the questions, read through the section again to refresh your understanding before moving on.

References

Allitt Inquiry (1991) *Independent Inquiry relating to Deaths and Injuries on the Children's Ward at Grantham and Kesteven General Hospital during the Period February to April 1991*. HMSO, London.

Aston University, (1999) *Team Working and Effectiveness in Health Care*. Aston Business School, Birmingham.

Barton, R. (1967) *Sans Everything: A Case to Answer*. Nelson, London.

Bristol Royal Infirmary Inquiry, (2001), *Learning from Bristol: The Report of the Public Inquiry into Children's Heart Surgery at the Bristol Royal Infirmary 1984–1995*. The Stationery Office, London. Available from www.bristol-inquiry.org.uk/final_report/index.htm.

Cabinet Office (1999) *Modernising Government*. The Stationery Office, London.

Cayton, H. (2005) Some Thoughts on Medical Professionalism and Regulation. Conference speech, ASME Defining and Developing Professionalism Conference, 28 April.

Corben, S. and Rosen, R. (2005), *Self Management for Long term Conditions: Patients' Perspectives on the Way Ahead*. Kings Fund, London.

Coulter, A. (2002) *The Autonomous Patient: Ending Paternalism in Medical Care*. The Nuffield Trust, The Stationery Office, London.

Department of Health (1996) *The Patient's Charter and You: A Charter for England*. The Stationery Office, London.

Department of Health, (2000), *The NHS Plan: A Plan for Investment, a Plan for Reform*. The Stationery Office, London.

Department of Health (2001a) *The Bristol Royal Infirmary Inquiry*. The Stationery Office, London.

Department of Health (2001b) *The Expert Patient: A New Approach to Chronic Disease Management for the 21st Century*. The Stationery Office, London.

Department of Health, (2003) *Building on the Best: Choice, Responsiveness and Equity in the NHS*. The Stationery Office, London.

Department of Health, (2004) *The NHS Improvement Plan*. HMSO, London.

Department of Health (2005a) *'Now I Feel Tall': What a Patient-led NHS Feels Like*. HMSO, London.

Department of Health (2005b) *Creating a Patient-led NHS: Delivering the NHS Improvement Plan*. DoH, London.

Dickson, A. (2004) *Difficult Conversations*. Piatkus, London.

Garland, G. (2006) Back to the Floor. *Health Service Journal*, **116**(5988): 31.

Griffiths Report (1983) *NHS Management Inquiry Report*, DHSS, London.

Health and Social Care Act 2001. HSMO, London.

Henley Management College (2005) *Evaluation of the Leadership at the Point of Care Programme*. Henley Management College, Greenlands.

Jay, D (1937) *The Socialist Case*. Faber and Faber, London.

Klein, R. (2001) *The New Politics of the NHS*. Prentice Hall, London.

Kotter, J. and Cohen, D. (2002) *The Heart of Change*. HBS Press, Harvard.

Morrison, B. (2006) I said to the nurse, please feed her. *The Guardian* (7 Jan.).

National Consumer Council (2004) *Making Public Services Personal: A New Compact for Public Services*. NCC, London.

Picker Institute (2005) *Is the NHS Getting Better or Worse?* Picker Institute, Europe.

Shipman Inquiry (2004) *Fifth Report – Safeguarding Patients: Lessons from the Past – Proposals for the Future*. HSMO, London.

Timmins, N. (1995) *The Five Giants: A Biography of the Welfare State*. HarperCollins, London.

World Health Organization. (2006) *Working Together for Health*. WHO, Geneva.

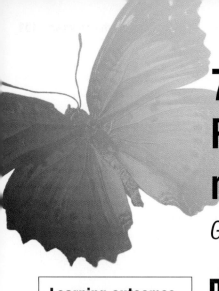

7
Patient-centred management

Gayle Garland

Learning outcomes

By the end of this chapter you should be able to:

★ Describe the difference between patient-centred management and managing the patient

★ Examine your personal experience of power and empowerment and how that experience influences your relationship with the patient

★ Give examples of ways to solicit and respond to feedback from patients

★ Develop strategies for handling challenging patient situations such as dissatisfaction.

Introduction

Every encounter by a patient with the health care system has two dimensions: the events, and the experience. The events are the objective details of the encounter, and the experience is the subjective or personal meaning attached to the encounter. Take, for example, having to wait past your appointment time to see your GP. One patient may be annoyed because the delay is making her late for picking up her children from the childminder. Another patient may be anxious and impatient because he is awaiting important test results. Still another patient may be quite relaxed and calm, the waiting time giving her a chance to finish an interesting article in a magazine. These patients are faced with the same events, yet they have very different experiences. Each person will remember the experience with more intensity than the event. The actual length of delay is not particularly important; it is the meaning attached to the delay that creates the experience. Meaning is the important ingredient in experience.

Event + Meaning = Experience

Over to you

Below are a number of meanings that could be attributed to a delay at your GP surgery.

- The office staff should know how long the doctor usually takes with a patient; they must be booking the appointments too close together.
- The office staff book appointments correctly; it's the GP that ignores the schedule.

- The office staff do a difficult job well; a few minutes delay is no problem.
- The office staff don't care if I have to wait.
- The GP doesn't care if he keeps me waiting.
- The GP is too busy.
- The GP is told by the government that she can only allow 10 minutes per patient. It's not her fault that the appointments take longer; it's the government's fault I have to wait.
- The GP talks too much; she should get on with the job and stop chatting.
- If I were paying for this appointment, I certainly wouldn't sit here and take this.
- Other patients are so inconsiderate; they take as long as they want, not even caring that there is a waiting room full of people.
- What's the point of coming to appointments on time? I always have to wait. Next appointment, I'll come late and see how they like it.
- This is unusual. I have never known my GP to keep me waiting. She must be very busy.
- I don't mind waiting, it gives me a longer lunch break and my boss can't complain.

What other meanings might you attribute to the delay?

Keywords

Patient-centred management

Is a process of designing and delivering services that accommodate the needs, beliefs and preferences of each individual with a view to creating a good experience as judged by that individual

Having to wait past an appointment time can be interpreted in many different ways. Health care staff have a responsibility to manage not only the events on behalf of the patient, but also the experience. **Patient-centred management** involves designing health services that balance the events and the experience, to create a satisfying result in the eyes of the patient.

Managing the patient

Modernisation of the NHS means moving from a profession-centred model to a patient-centred model (see Chapter 6). Under the profession-centred model of health care, the purpose of management activity is to fit the patient into the system. Health services were originally designed around doctors and hospitals so that a consultant could see as many patients as possible without having to travel. Ideally, consultants could attend clinic, do surgery, complete hospital rounds, and teach students all within the same four walls. The patients were managed with the intention of making the system work most efficiently. Patients would sometimes spend hours waiting for their turn to be seen.

One of the results of the profession-centred model is that patients find themselves being passed from professional to professional and from service to service. The NHS was founded on the principle that everyone should have equal access to health care based on need, not ability to pay. That means that all patients needing surgery, who are comparably ill, are

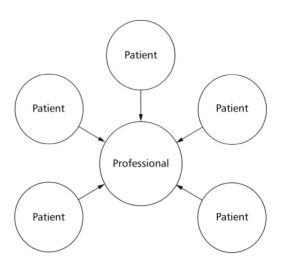

Profession-centred services

equally entitled to have their surgery. The problem comes when there are more patients needing surgery than can immediately be accommodated. The solution has been to prioritise surgery (and some other services) on a first-come, first-served basis. This is one of the most common and most accepted forms of prioritisation; we see it every day at the bus stop. In fact, in the earlier days of the NHS, relatively little complaint was heard from the public. Waiting for service was accepted as part of the price to be paid for universal access to health care (Rivett, 2006).

Here is a typical referral process for a person with osteoarthritis of the hip in a profession-centred model of health care.

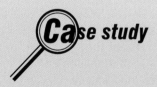

Osteoarthritis of the hip progressing to hip replacement

A patient visits a GP with groin pain. The GP diagnoses muscular problems or mild arthritis and recommends pain relievers and anti-inflammatory medication.

The patient presents several months later at the GP surgery with progressing pain and now has a limp. The diagnosis of osteoarthritis of the hip is made; medication is adjusted, and the patient is encouraged to stay active. The patient presents again to the GP with increasing pain and disability. A referral is made to orthopaedic services for assessment. The patient waits. The patient is seen by a physiotherapist: the first step in the orthopaedic assessment process. The patient is told that hip-replacement surgery will eventually be needed; however, for now, advice is given and walking aids are provided.

The patient continues to see a physiotherapist and a GP for pain control and maintenance of mobility. The physiotherapist decides that the condition is progressing and therapy is no longer the treatment of choice. Referral is made to the orthopaedic surgeon. The patient waits. The orthopaedic surgeon assesses the patient and recommends surgery. The patient is placed on the surgeon's list. The patient waits up to six months. A surgical date is offered. The patient waits. A pre-operative assessment is done and, if fit, the patient is cleared for surgery. The patient has surgery.

- How would you rate this experience in terms of patient-centred care?
- How would you feel if this was you?
- How would you manage this system to make it more patient centred?

Patient-centred management

Put simply, the most important principle underpinning patient-centred management and patient-centred service design and delivery is how it will meet the needs of the patients using the service.

Modernisation in the health service is no different from the modernisation that has occurred over the last 20 years in other services, both public and commercial. Take the banking industry as an example. It is not too many years since banks were only open a limited number of hours (10.00 a.m. until 3.00 p.m. – known colloquially as 'bankers' hours') and customers had to fit in with that service. During the 1980s and 1990s, life became increasingly complex for the public. Many people worked away from their homes and were not able to do their banking locally during bankers' hours. Banks responded by opening local branches to customers from other branches, but that did not satisfy people for long. The public began to expect even more from their banks, such as the ability to obtain cash withdrawals and statements at all hours. Banks met these demands by closing local branches and replacing them with a network of electronic services (cash machines and online and telephone banking). For many customers, the changes in banking were welcome, as they provided increased flexibility and easy access.

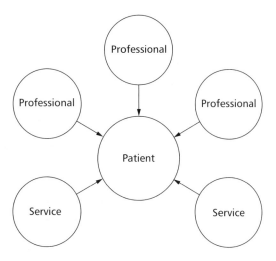

Patient-centred services

As with any fundamental change in service, not every bank customer was happy with the new services. Some missed the personal attention that they had received when they went into their local branch. Those unable to travel and with no access to computers were cut off from access to banking services altogether.

When providing health care services, we are often challenged to perform a delicate balancing act between the preferences of a particular person and the needs of the many. For example, if we were to allow one patient to stay as long as they wished in hospital, the treatment of others could, as a result, be delayed.

What patients want

Whilst there may be differences between what each *individual* wants from the health service, the following eight factors were identified by the Picker Institute's (2005) survey as those that patients *as a whole* consider most important (see also Chapter 6, p. 134):

- fast access to reliable health care
- effective treatment delivered by trusted professionals
- involvement in decisions and respect for preferences
- clear, comprehensive information and support for self-care
- attention to physical and environmental needs
- emotional support, empathy and respect
- involvement of, and support for, family and carers
- continuity of care and smooth transitions.

One way to become a more patient-centred manager would be to use the above factors as a benchmark against which services are compared.

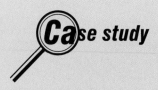
Case study

Patient-centred services

A dermatology service has a walk-in clinic to screen moles and other lesions for skin cancers. Any GP can refer a patient simply by providing a letter for the patient to take to the clinic. The clinic is open on Wednesday mornings, and there is no need to make an appointment. When the patient is seen at the clinic, the skin lesion is assessed, and, if appropriate, removed. The tissue removed is sent to the lab for analysis and the patient is given an appointment to return in four weeks for the results. The results are also sent to the GP who made the referral, with a copy of any follow-up instructions.

- How many of the eight factors most important to patients does this service meet? How could this service be changed to make it even more patient centred?

Table 7.1 Comparison of profession-centred and patient-centred care/services

Profession-centred care/service	Patient-centred care/service
Serviced designed by professionals	Services designed by patients
Business hours	All hours
Decisions made by professionals	Decisions made by patients
Patients are passed from service to service, professional to professional	Services are moved closer to the patients or coordinated to create a 'one-stop' service whenever possible
Professional knows best	Patient knows best
Gives advice	Informs and discusses

Becoming more patient centred

Becoming more patient centred challenges us to put ourselves in the patient's shoes and to examine closely two things: the events and the experience. These are flip sides of the same coin and equate to a balance between what you do and how you do it.

Reflective activity

Think about these two contrasting services.

1. Autobirth: a new machine has been invented to manage childbirth in a 'humane and efficient' way. Close to the end of pregnancy, the Autobirth analyser is attached to the abdomen of the pregnant woman. The analyser determines exactly the best time for childbirth and alerts the woman 24 hours in advance. Autobirth also sends a wireless email to the birthing centre reserving a platform. At the appointed time, the woman is admitted to the birthing centre, with the Autobirth analyser sending a security code enabling entry. The woman is directed by computer screen to her platform and positions herself, based on the pressure-sensitive pads on the platform. Once she is properly aligned, the computer anaesthetises her with just the right amount of drugs. The child is delivered either by caesarean section (with micro scar repair) or rapid vaginal extraction (as determined by Autobirth) and the mother is revived. The child is auto-screened, auto-wrapped and placed in her arms on the platform. Autobirth sends her partner a text (he has the option to view the birth on his mobile), telling him to pick her up. The procedure takes less than an hour.

2. Earthbirth: a natural birth option is available. Close to the end of the pregnancy, your personal attendant moves in with you to start the birth preparation process. You spend every waking hour with her, meditating, exercising and preparing. When she believes that you are ready, the two of you and your partner leave the house and move into the birth cave.

There you assist in other births and learn natural pain management. When you go into labour, the other women and their partners surround you and help as they can. No machines are used; no medicines are available; there are no phones; there is not even electricity. There is no way to contact the outside world, as this is an immersion experience. After the birth, you and your partner are free to return home on the Birth Cave Express that arrives and leaves once a week.

- Which service would you choose and why?
- What parts of each service are attractive to you?

This reflection is intended to illustrate that neither an efficiency-based service nor a relationship-based service is sufficient on its own. Patient experience is made up of a subtle mix of ingredients.

The following eight factors were identified by nurses and patients as keys to creating confidence in care (Department of Health, 2006, in press):

- the physical environment
- the social and cultural environment
- the provision of personalised care
- caring *for* patients and significant others (technical and cultural competence)
- caring *about* patients and significant others (spiritual and interpersonal competence)
- resources, organisation and delivery of service
- collective responsibility for the service, performance and quality
- caring for and about each other (collective concern and consideration).

Evidence base

The document *Confidence in Caring* will be published in 2006 and be available via the publications page on the Department of Health website (www.dh.gov.uk). We recommend that you read it.

You will have noticed that there is overlap with some of the factors from the Picker Institute's survey (2005). In particular, both studies identify a mixture of service and relationship factors that work together to create the patient experience.

Patient-centred service management

The public are increasingly accustomed to seamless service in their lives. When that seamless service occurs, we hardly notice. Every day, thousands of people go to the airport, check in, catch flights and arrive at destinations within a few minutes of the scheduled arrival time. The public expect that health care services will evolve to have the same efficiency and simplicity. The following are areas to attend to when managing patient events.

Physical environment

The look and feel of the physical space in which services are offered are important elements in patient-centred management. Disarray, disorder and untidiness convey a lack of attention and concern to the public, and can lead to anxiety and distrust.

Imagine walking into a home that you were thinking of buying and finding dirty marks on the walls, stained toilets, and clutter on every surface. How would you feel about buying the house? Would you want to live there?

Paying attention to the physical surroundings is seldom a priority with staff; however, environmental factors can have an enormous effect on patients, as the remarks in the box below illustrate.

Patients' comments

- When I was in hospital, I had nothing to do all day. I used to notice things like the flowers that were past their prime on the windowsill. I wished someone would throw them away.
- The shower in our room was very old and looked like it hadn't been cleaned in ages. There is no way I would use it.
- I had to sit outside radiography in a patient gown in the hall with everyone walking past. I was so embarrassed.

Reflective activity

Look around your clinical area as if you are seeing it for the first time.
- If it were a hotel, what rating would you give it?
- What is inviting about your area?
- What is distracting and concerning about your area?

Location and organisation of services

Moving services closer to the patient is not always possible. Large diagnostic equipment such as X-ray machines and MRI scanners are difficult to move and need special conditions and trained technicians to operate them. Patients understand these constraints. What patients want is that, wherever possible, their circumstances are considered and adjustments are made to accommodate them.

Pre-operative visits that involve laboratory tests, X-rays and assessment by professionals should be organised on the same day and as close together as possible. If it is necessary for the patient to visit more than one department, it is best if they are escorted. The need for assistance with mobility should be anticipated so that people are available to help. It is useful if staff ask about special needs when clinic appointments are made so that these can be more easily accommodated.

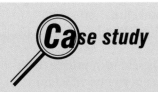

Alzheimer's disease

Mrs Grey was recently referred to a consultant clinic. She is a full-time carer for her husband who has Alzheimer's disease. The only day of the week that she has respite care for her husband is Tuesday. She was sent an appointment for Thursday, the only day of the week that the consultant does new-patient assessments at that site. She phoned up to see what arrangements can be made.

- Which of the following options would you choose to resolve the situation?
- Which is the most patient centred?
  - Offer her an appointment with another consultant who has clinic on a Tuesday.
  - Offer to let her bring her husband with her, and you will take care of him whilst she has her appointment.
  - Offer to work with the respite services to cover her clinic appointment.
  - Talk to the consultant about setting up a special arrangement on a Tuesday.

You may have spotted the trick in this case study. The answer is that whichever solution best suits Mrs Grey is the most patient centred. Asking the patient what she prefers is always a good starting point. Health professionals are often afraid to ask a patient what they want for fear that the request will be unreasonable or impossible to meet. The reality is that most patients are reasonable and most requests can be honoured. Even when the patient's request cannot be fully satisfied, knowing what the person wants is a more authentic starting point and allows for a better solution to be achieved.

Patient-centred experience management

One of the most important lessons from the Confidence in Caring project (Department of Health, 2006, in press) is that patients notice everything, all the time. Staff seldom realise just how much patients hear and see or the impact that those experiences have on the patient.

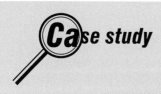

Personal experience

As part of a pre-operative assessment, I was asked to come in for an echocardiogram. I arrived 10 minutes early and was shown to a seat in the waiting area where I was the only patient. Four staff members were sitting at a table in the staffroom discussing the trust's plans to implement the new 'choose and book' appointment system. They were all agreed that they would not be able to accommodate the new system without the addition of a full-time secretary. They did not like the system because it took control of appointments away from them. The discussion went on for 15 minutes as I waited for my test to be done (for 5 of those minutes, they were talking in the waiting area where I was sitting, and my presence was not acknowledged).

Finally, one of the staff members acknowledged me, smiled and invited me into the treatment room. She went on to explain the procedure fully, protect my dignity during the test, reassure me that the test result was normal, and answer my questions thoroughly and appropriately.

Imagine yourself in my shoes during the two contrasting experiences described above.

- Which of the following statements best reflects the beliefs underlying my behaviour in the waiting room?
- Which statement best reflects the beliefs underlying my behaviour in the treatment room?

  - Professionals are my equal. They are knowledgeable and experienced in health matters, and I have a right to be fully informed and involved along the way. We share responsibility for this experience.

  - These people aren't concerned about me; all they are worried about is how this new system will affect their work. I'll just sit here pretending to be invisible until someone says something. I wouldn't want to upset them; they are in control here. I need to keep them on my side, or they might just make things worse for me.

  - I'm the customer here; they shouldn't be chatting about work while I'm waiting. I have the right to good service. After all, my wages pay their salaries, they work for me.

We are often unaware that there is an underlying set of beliefs, values and experience that affects our behaviour. Imagine for a moment that you are a new student undertaking your first clinical placement. How do you feel: in control, knowledgeable, capable and confident; or scared, vulnerable, out of place and ignorant? Chances are that you were feeling closer to the second set of descriptors, and would spend your clinical time hoping that nobody would ask you any questions that you could not answer. The idea that anyone would let you work with the patients was frightening; you may have felt that you presented more of a risk to the patient than a help.

It may surprise you to learn that, as a rule, patients feel relatively powerless in relation to health care staff, even students (Oshry, 1995).

> ### ☞ *Over to you*
>
> Take a few minutes to jot down the factors that contribute to the likelihood that patients will feel relatively less powerful and in control than the health professionals treating them?
>
> - How could you change some of these factors to help the patient feel more comfortable in a clinical situation?

Working toward empowerment

Empowerment is a concept that is defined differently depending on the situation. In the context of work, empowerment usually relates to giving authority to an individual to undertake a particular responsibility. Doctors are empowered by law to prescribe medicines. Managers are empowered by their employer to make decisions about spending their budget. Health care professionals are empowered by virtue of their professional knowledge to make recommendations about appropriate treatment in a clinical situation.

When we talk about empowering the patient, it usually means enabling the patient to participate more effectively in their own care, should they wish to do so, by building their knowledge and confidence. Empowerment can extend to enabling patients or members of the public to participate in the planning, evaluation and design of health services for other people

The way that one individual feels in relation to another influences their behaviour. Let me give you an example. Most adults relate to school-aged children in a predictable way. Because school-aged children are less experienced in life, less knowledgeable and less aware, they can make poor decisions and behave in a way that is unsafe for them. Adults respond to this lack of capability by protecting the child and limiting their choices. In other words, adults exercise control over children in an effort to protect and teach them.

It is not only adults and children that fall into this behaviour pattern. Whenever we see the other person as less capable than us, we have a tendency to exercise control over them. Think again of the circumstances of your first clinical placement. You saw yourself as inexperienced and less knowledgeable compared with the qualified professionals and the instructors around you, so you deferred to them in relation to decisions and allowed yourself to be directed. Your giving over of control to those other professionals was appropriate, based on your clinical capabilities.

The subtle dynamics of power are present in every interaction, but, most of the time, power dynamics are not a part of our awareness. (Oshry, 1995). We subconsciously place ourselves in a more powerful, less powerful or relatively equal relationship depending on the situation. Here is another example.

One of your neighbours is a police officer. Your children play together and you invite each other to barbecues and other social events. You look after each other's house when you are away. Is the relationship here one of equals or one in which one of you is more powerful?

You are driving home in a hurry to pick up your children. You are stopped for speeding, and, to your horror, the officer who stopped you is your neighbour. The officer issues a speeding fine, and you go on your way home. Is this is a relationship of equals? If not, who is the more powerful and why?

The following week you are on duty in the A&E. Your neighbour is admitted with abdominal pain and vomiting and is diagnosed with appendicitis. You take care of her until she goes to theatre. Is this a relationship of equals? If not, who is the more powerful and why?

Whether or not you are aware of it, how you treat people in a given situation is influenced by how powerful you feel in relation to them. Whether you see them as capable or vulnerable, knowledgeable or ignorant, calm or anxious will affect the way that you relate to them.

The profession-centred model of health care arose during a time when health care professionals had unique knowledge, privileged information, status and position. Patients were perceived as ignorant and many professionals saw them as incapable, which led to the belief that professionals should make decisions on behalf of the patient. Even now, health professionals still have a formal power advantage over patients owing to their education, qualification and experience. However, the differences between patients and professionals are diminishing.

Patient-centred care is an attempt to level the field between patients and professionals. The patient-centred model assumes that patients are better informed, and more capable of self-determination than ever before, and that beliefs, experiences, knowledge, and preferences should be respected. Patient-centred care means that the professional is willing to relinquish the power advantage by fully informing, involving and respecting the patient.

Reflective activity

Think back to at least three recent experiences with patients. Read the following statements.

1. This patient is my equal. He is capable, intelligent and experienced and should be fully involved in every aspect of his care. We share responsibilities: I am responsible for sharing my expertise, and he is responsible for weighing the information and choosing the course of action that is best for him.

2. I'm going to have to take responsibility for this patient. He has little knowledge or experience of his condition. He is not coping very well, and I'm afraid he'll make a bad decision without my guidance. It is important that I take a strong lead until he is better able to manage.

3. This patient is impossible! I have advised, cajoled and told, but he hasn't listened to a word I've said. I don't know why he bothers to consult me when he does what he pleases anyway. At least I can honestly say I've done my job.

- Which of the statements represents your feelings about the patient in the three recent experiences that you recalled?

- In each example, what is the health professional's power relationship with the patient?

Patient-centred management of experience centres on moving the relationship between the professional and the patient from one that is unequal to one that is equal. That is not to say that equality of relationship is appropriate in all circumstances. Emergencies require professionals to exercise control over the situation until the patient is again able to participate fully. When people are very ill or emotionally distressed, it may be necessary to make decisions for them.

There has been a tendency in the past, however, to continue to exercise control over patients when it is no longer appropriate. One of the fields of practice where this has been most apparent is mental health. Until fairly recently, patients with enduring mental illness were committed to asylums, and, once admitted, the assumption was that they would remain there for life. The policy of committing mentally ill people was done with the best of intentions: in the asylum the patient was housed, fed, and protected. The mental health services could be described as a benevolent surrogate parent to these unfortunate people.

Though well intended, this policy was flawed. Contrary to conventional wisdom, most mentally ill people were not content to be looked after in these institutions for life: most wanted to participate in life as much as they were capable. This meant that the mental health services would have to move to a position where they were less parental and more equal in respect of the patients they served.

In some circumstances, health professionals and managers have been reluctant to relinquish the parental role. Consider the following situation, taking a moment to reflect on the question posed at the end.

Reflective activity

You are a district nurse. You have been visiting a patient for a long time to assist her in her diabetes management. Philosophically and practically, you work hard to achieve independence for your patients. There are other patients waiting for service and you are feeling stretched to provide what is needed.

Each time that you have tried to get this patient to take more responsibility for her own care, and therefore pave the way for the service to be withdrawn, she becomes tearful and says, 'Oh, no, nurse, I couldn't possibly manage on my own. Can't you continue to see me?'

This is a difficult situation for the district nurse. One of the main reasons why people go into the health professions is that they want to help others. This patient clearly wants the nurse to keep visiting; on some level, the nurse feels good about the visits as well. Most people like to be needed and to feel wanted; nurses are no different in that respect.

If the nurse withdraws services, the patient is not likely to cope for long, and the nurse may feel as if she is abandoning her responsibilities. If she keeps the patient on services, she is aware that she is denying service to others and is increasing this patient's tendency to dependency. The dilemma arises when the nurse asks herself, 'Which choice represents patient-centred management?'

The answer is that neither moving her off service, nor keeping her on service is the patient-centred choice at this moment. To be truly patient centred, the nurse must determine exactly what need her visits are fulfilling and help the patient to fulfil that need elsewhere. In that way, the patient is empowered to manage her own care and to meet her needs without continuing dependency on the district nurse. Then the nurse can ethically move the patient off services without in any way disadvantaging the patient.

What may be getting in the way of this nurse's effective management of the situation is her underlying subconscious belief. The nurse and the patient have been in a long-standing, unequal relationship, and neither nurse nor patient can imagine a relationship of equality. The patient continues to give control to the nurse, and the nurse continues to hold control.

In this situation, the nurse must take the first step in moving the relationship forward. Consider the following reflection/action steps (adapted from *Difficult Conversations* by Ann Dickson, 2004):

1. The starting point is the nurse's recognition that she is not being patient centred in her care; she is creating a long-term dependency that is not in the interests of the patient.

2. The nurse should reflect on what benefit she is gaining from the relationship with the patient (friendship, a sense of being needed, pleasant conversation, cups of tea, easy predictable work) and plan for satisfying that need elsewhere.

3. Plan to speak to the patient. If needed, role-play the situation with a colleague. The nurse needs to approach the patient as an equal, with the expectation that something positive will come out of the discussion.

4. Use the following as a guide to the conversation. These steps ensure that the nurse makes every effort to build equality and joint responsibility into the discussion.

   - Tell the patient how you are feeling about the situation: for example, 'Mrs H, I have been seeing you for a year now, and I now feel that you are very capable of managing your diabetes care and I think it is appropriate that my visits stop. I would be sad about that because I really enjoy visiting you. I am concerned that we seem to be stuck, with neither of us moving on the way we should.'

   - Tell the patient what you want: 'Mrs H, I want to work out a way for my visits to decrease and eventually stop, in a way that doesn't upset you, or put you at risk.'

   - Ask for her cooperation and ideas: 'I need your help to work out the plan. What are your ideas?'

5. Ideally, the patient will respond as an equal and work with the nurse to solve the problem. However, it is not uncommon for people to want to maintain their unequal relationship. If this happens, restate your intention to work together to draw up a plan for the visits to stop, in a way that is satisfactory to both parties. Give the patient time to think about it, and promise to keep seeing them until something can be worked out. This statement of beneficial intention will often succeed in moving the relationship to a more equal footing in the long run.

Listening to patients

One of the biggest challenges facing health care organisations is the meaningful involvement of patients. Policy changes have helped organisations to move in the right direction, but policy alone is not enough. Patients and the public must be helped towards a feeling of greater equality in order for patient-centred management to become fully implemented.

As we explored in the last section, it is common for patients to feel relatively powerless in relation to the professionals around them. There are many reasons for this. Professionals have more clinical knowledge and more information about the health care system; they know people inside the system who can help and guide them; they have better health, higher status and often operate from their offices, thereby having 'home court' advantage. Professionals also have direct control over patients, such as the ability to prescribe medication, make a referral, or to authorise surgery or other treatment. Under the Mental Health Act, professionals even have the right to hold people against their will.

In view of this apparent imbalance of power, it is not hard to imagine why it can be difficult to find out how the patient really feels. If your doctor has the power to withdraw medicines that you rely on, are you likely to tell her that you do not like her attitude? If the consultant decides who goes on the waiting list, are you likely to question his clinical skill? Being in an unequal relationship causes the weaker person to be cautious about speaking up.

Several mechanisms have been used to tap into the patient's and public's experience of health services. Large-scale surveys of public opinion have been undertaken and published, such as the Picker Institute survey mentioned previously in this chapter and in Chapter 6 (see pages 134 and 154). These large-scale surveys are a good representation of the consensus of the public's views and are quite useful as principles against which to benchmark current practice.

Integral to the inspections conducted by the Healthcare Commission is evidence that the trust is listening to and incorporating patient views into trust policies. Most trusts now conduct some form of patient audit, and you might be asked to participate, or to review the results of an audit.

Most audits of patient views are taken after the patient leaves hospital. This is done in an attempt to get more honest feedback, as patients who are in hospital often feel too vulnerable to speak up. One difficulty with asking people about their experience after the fact is that the patient has gone home, and you may not have the opportunity to make amends.

Complaints and compliments

Every health care organisation has a procedure for dealing with compliments and complaints. Compliments are often logged and used as evidence of satisfactory patient experiences. Complaints are handled in a more formal way.

The chief executive of the trust has the ultimate accountability for responding to any complaint. Usually, the complaint is received by the chief executive's office and is then passed along to a staff member to investigate. If the complaint is about a specific service or ward, the person in charge of that area is likely to be asked to look into the matter. The investigation often includes contact with the complainant and interviews with all staff involved. Notes are reviewed and any incident reports are read. Once a full account of the circumstances is compiled, a letter is sent back to the complainant. If the complainant is satisfied with the response, no further action is needed. If dissatisfied, the complainant can refer the situation on to the strategic health authority or, if the concern is about a clinical professional, they can write to the licensing body of that profession. (Department of Health, 2004a)

Learning from complaints

Although the formal process of responding to complaints is important, the real learning from complaints comes from the way in which complaints are handled by professionals. Patient-centred management involves really listening to the patient's experience even though it may feel painful. To hear yourself described as abrupt or rude, or to hear your colleagues referred to as uncaring, can be difficult. It is, however, the patient's experience: the meaning that they have attributed to the events.

Instead of reacting on an emotional level, it is more helpful to consider the events and the circumstances to see if anything could have changed the experience. Some of the actions below can be useful when events cannot be changed.

- **Unexpected delay**. Offer an apology for the delay, a short explanation as to the reason for the delay, and a realistic estimate of the new time frame. Where possible, offer alternatives such as another appointment time or a more comfortable waiting area; make the offer of a cup of tea or a brief chat.

- **Lack of information or a delay in reaching someone**. Offer an apology followed by an account of the efforts that are being made to find the information or locate the person. Be honest about the situation and make a commitment to keep trying.

- **Lack of courtesy or rudeness**. Hopefully this will not happen too often, but, when it does, the matter needs to be handled sensitively. Apologise for the upset experienced. Do not justify the other person's actions, or explain. Simply apologise and offer to help.

Being open

The National Patient Safety Agency has been very active in studying and publishing best practice in working with patients. One of the most difficult situations in which a health professional could find themselves is when a patient is seriously harmed or has died as a result of a patient-safety event. Under a profession-centred model of care, information was withheld from the patient and family in an effort to protect the health professional and the health service. Unfortunately, the effect of this policy was just the opposite with patients and carers taking out a law suit because they have not received any information or an apology from the health care team or organisation.

Being Open (National Patient Safety Agency, 2005) argues that there is evidence to support the desire for openness by patients. A survey of 8000 people in the UK, 400 of whom had experienced a patient-safety incident, revealed that they wanted the NHS to respond in the following ways:

- 34% wanted an apology or explanation
- 23% wanted an inquiry into the cause
- 17% wanted support for coping with the consequences
- 11% wanted financial compensation
- 6% wanted disciplinary action
- 9% wanted another response or did not respond.

The findings of the Australian National Open Disclosure Project (2003) were very similar. It found that patients would like:

- to be told about an incident that affects them
- an acknowledgement of the distress they experience
- a sincere and compassionate statement of regret for the distress caused
- a clear statement of what is going to happen
- a plan of what can be done medically to repair or redress the harm done.

The National Patient Safety Agency (2005) went on to recommend a process for communicating with patients following a clinical event that causes harm. The following 10 principles underpin the process of communication and are recommended to form the basis of local practice.

1. **The principle of acknowledgement**. All incidents should be acknowledged and reported as soon as they are discovered.
2. **The principle of truthfulness, timeliness and clarity of communication**. Patients and their families should be given a step-by-step account of the events, delivered openly and as soon as practicable after the event.
3. **The principle of apology**. There should be a sincere expression of regret for the harm that has occurred, verbally and in writing.
4. **The principle of recognising patient and carer expectations**. Patients and family reasonably expect a face-to-face meeting in which they are fully informed.
5. **Principle of professional support**. Professionals should be supported to report incidents.
6. **Principle of risk management and systems improvement**. Openness is part of an integrated approach to patient safety.
7. **Principle of multidisciplinary responsibility**. The local policy on openness applies to all staff.
8. **Principle clinical governance**. There should be learning from the experience.

9. **Principle of confidentiality**. Details of the patient-safety incident should at all times remain confidential. Sharing of any detail beyond the clinical team involved should only be done on a need-to-know basis and, where possible, with permission of the individual involved.

10. **Principle of continuity of care**. Patients should continue to receive treatment and care.

Two of these principles, in particular, are a basis for good practice in patient-centred management in a more general sense.

One is the principle of truthfulness, timeliness and clarity of communication. This principle was illustrated in the activity on page 163, in which you were asked to reflect on the case of a district nurse who was trying to move her patient off services and towards greater independence. How would you apply the principle to the following situation?

Reflective activity

A patient phones you up and is very angry that she has not yet received an appointment to see the consultant. She is in pain and having trouble taking care of her small children. She is demanding an immediate appointment or she will file a complaint. How do you respond?

Abiding by the principle of truthfulness, timeliness and clarity of communication, you would:

1. Apologise for the wait.

2. Acknowledge that it sounds as if the situation is getting particularly difficult for her.

3. Explain that you will find out immediately when it is likely that her appointment will come up.

4. Offer to phone her back within the hour to set up the appointment or to redirect her back to her GP for re-evaluation.

The other is the principle of recognising patient and carer expectations. It is not always easy to know what people expect. We have survey data that suggest that patients want good service (convenience and responsiveness similar to what is available elsewhere) and a satisfying experience. But how can you find out what an individual actually expects?

> ## Reflective activity
>
> You work on a day surgery unit, and you are alarmed to see Mr S come in with a large suitcase for what should be a hernia repair as a day case. How will you approach the situation?

The best approach is to be open and direct. One model is to give effective feedback followed by a question to explore expectations.

> Mr S, you seem to have brought a very big case with you.
> It makes me wonder how long you were expecting to stay.

Helping patients and the public to participate more effectively

Helping patients to participate more fully in their own health care and in the design of health services is not easy. There are practical obstacles to overcome as well as establishing a relationship in which the patient feels sufficiently empowered to want to participate.

Practical barriers to participation

One of the most common barriers to patient participation or public involvement is the way that health services are structured. Meetings and appointments are often scheduled between 9.00 a.m. and 5.00 p.m., Mondays to Fridays. This could make it very difficult for a patient with a job or care responsibilities to participate.

Most of the time, the patient has to travel to the professional's office or to the organisation to participate. This is particularly true when the patient is invited to meet with a group of professionals or managers. Travel can be expensive; and not all trusts pay patients to participate. There are, in any case, strict limits to the amount that a trust can pay a patient or member of the public for their participation, and this can cause hardship for some people. Physical disability can also get in the way of participation, as some areas are difficult to access without help.

Patients and members of the public may not have access to the Internet or other sources of reputable information that would help them to be better informed and therefore more willing to participate on an equal footing. Few health service facilities offer Internet access to the public although most public libraries now provide Internet services free of charge. Not knowing how to access information, on the Internet or in print, can be another barrier to members of the public.

Overcoming these practical barriers challenges health professionals and organisations to work differently. *Getting over the Wall: How the NHS is Improving the Patient's Experience* (Department of Health, 2004b) has some excellent case studies. Here are some examples:

- Brent Primary Care Trust wanted to get the opinions of learning disability users so it went to the local day centres that the service users were attending.
- Hammersmith Hospitals NHS Trust held a patients' panel in the evening at Charing Cross Hospital where a light supper was provided.
- West of Cornwall Primary Care Trust wanted feedback from travellers so it enlisted one of the travellers to gather the views of other travellers and to bring those to a travellers' forum consisting of health visitors, social services, travellers and a travellers' education officer.
- Hull and East Riding Stroke Services worked with a local group of stroke survivors, Strokewatch, to implement a number of changes.

Personal barriers to participation

Some factors that can increase the feelings of inequality between professionals and patients need to be considered. Effective working relationships are much more likely to evolve when patients and the public feel understood and valued by health professionals. Several actions can be taken by health professionals to build a more effective relationship of equity and empowerment with patients.

- Understand your own values, beliefs and preferences. The patient is not the only one who has values and beliefs. Each one of us comes with a collection of personal attributes that affects the way we respond to any situation. Let me give you a personal example. During a student placement, I was assigned to sit with a woman who was experiencing auditory hallucinations and see if I could engage her in simple conversation. After about 10 minutes, I was unsuccessful in getting her to talk. Not quite knowing what to do, I attempted to make eye contact by moving my face directly in front of hers. She responded by shrieking in horror and running for the door. I was frightened and embarrassed. That experience caused me to doubt my ability to work with similar patients, and I have always been a bit wary of being assigned to this type of care.
- Develop a familiarity with the cultural values, health beliefs, customs and practices of the ethnic, cultural and religious groups served by your department. This understanding will enable you to be more sensitive to the world view of people who are different from you. For example, if you want to attract local people from the Muslim community to a patient forum, it is probably best to avoid Friday.

- Ask how the patient prefers to be addressed; and tell them how you would like to be addressed. This is a simple suggestion but not without its practical difficulties. If the patient prefers to be addressed informally by their first name but you are addressed by your title, then inequality is reinforced. Are you willing for the patient to address you by your first name? Being on first-name basis with someone is a form of equality and familiarity that usually indicates trust, but is it appropriate?
- Determine the patient's level of fluency in English and arrange for a translator, if needed.
- Assure the patient of confidentiality and, whenever possible, arrange a private place to speak. In some cultures, rumours, jealousy, privacy and reputation are crucial issues, and these should be considered.
- Use a speech rate, tone, style and complexity that match the speech patterns of the patient. If the patient speaks slowly, it is usually best if you do the same. This not only improves understanding, but usually helps the other person to feel more comfortable.

This is not an exhaustive list of strategies; I'm sure that you can think of many more. The key to overcoming personal barriers to participation is to build a relationship of trust and equity with the person. This applies to patients with whom you are working professionally and to members of the public who are being invited to give feedback or to help improve services in your work area.

Principles of patient involvement

The following principles are important in achieving more patient involvement. They come from a document called *Strengthening Accountability – Involving Patients and the Public: Practice Guidance* (Department of Health, 2003).

1. **Make the best of what you have**. If you are routinely working with patients, they are a good source of information and experience. There is often no need to look further if your aim is to improve everyday patient experience.
2. **Plan well in advance**. It may be tempting to leap in and get on with it, but time spent planning is time well spent.
3. **Be honest**. Involvement can go wrong if people believe that they are being invited to explore a wide range of possibilities or to make decisions, when there are really only a couple of options that can be implemented. Be careful what you ask. If you ask patients if they would like a hot meal in the evening and that is not possible, you will be setting up a situation where the patients can end up feeling disregarded.

4. **Use the results**. Just asking for opinions is not enough. Patients and the public will expect changes as a result of their involvement.
5. **Take it seriously**. There needs to be genuine commitment, not a tick-box philosophy.

Reflective activity

Using the principles and strategies of patient-centred management that we have discussed so far, redesign your service (or a service you have recently worked in).

- How is the service accessed?
- How do patients and the public influence the service?
- What kind of relationships are there between patients and staff?
- Finally, using a metaphor, describe your redesigned service.

Summary

Patient-centred management involves incorporating the needs, beliefs and desires of the patients in everyday care, and the values, opinions and experience of patients and the public in designing services. Successfully transforming the health service away from the profession-centred model requires a change in beliefs, thinking and behaviour on behalf of the professionals and managers in the health service. Many of us came into health professions to help people, and for many that means taking care of people who are sick or injured. Too often, this has resulted in a parental style of behaviour, which disempowers the patient and keeps the professionals in control. The best of intentions have resulted in a long-standing, unequal relationship between the public and the health service.

As we move to a patient-led health service, there is a need for a relationship of equality and partnership that creates a shared responsibility between the service providers and the service users. As a health care professional working daily with patients, the way that you manage each patient contact will be either an example of managing the patient or one of patient-centred management. You are in control.

Rapid recap

Check your progress so far by working through each of the following questions:

1. Describe the difference between patient-centred management and managing the patient.
2. Describe five things that could turn a satisfactory event into a satisfying experience.
3. What actions can be taken to create a more equal perception of power between health care providers and patients?
4. Identify three conversational ways of moving a long-standing, unequal relationship between nurse and patient to one where the relationship is more equal and patient centred.
5. Identify three ways in which you could begin to include patients more in their care.

If you have difficulty with more than one of the questions, read through the section again to refresh your understanding before moving on.

References

Australian Council for Safety and Quality in Health Care (2003) *Open Disclosure Standard: A National Standard for Open Communication in Public and Private Hospitals, following an Adverse Event in Health Care*. Commonwealth of Australia, Sydney.

Department of Health (2003) *Strengthening Accountability – Involving Patients and the Public: Practice Guidance*. HMSO, London.

Department of Health (2004a) *How to Make a Complaint about the NHS*. HMSO, London.

Department of Health (2004b) *Getting over the Wall: How the NHS is Improving the Patient's Experience*. HMSO, London.

Department of Health. (2006, in press) *Confidence in Caring*.

Dickson, A. (2004) *Difficult Conversations*. Piatkus, London.

National Patient Safety Agency. (2005) *Being Open: Communicating Patient Safety Incidents with Patients and their Carers*. NPSA, London.

Oshry, B. (1995) *Seeing Systems: Unlocking the Mysteries of Organizational Life*. Berrett-Koehler, San Francisco.

Picker Institute (2005) *Is the NHS Getting Better or Worse?* Picker Institute, Europe.

Rivett, G. (2006) *Short NHS History*. www.nhshistory.net.

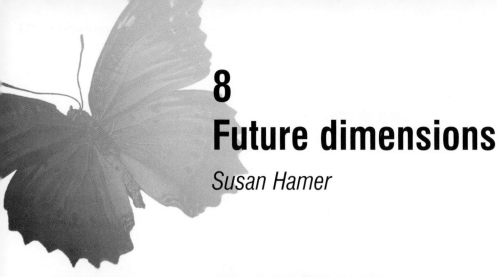

8
Future dimensions

Susan Hamer

Learning outcomes

By the end of this chapter you should be able to:

★ Understand the advantages of networks as an organisational form

★ List the characteristics of a community of practice

★ Understand some of the key characteristics associated with high-performance workplaces

★ Understand why ethical leadership and management is an important consideration for personal development

★ Understand the advantages of quiet leadership.

The future: a scenario

The alarm goes off, and I potter downstairs to get a coffee. As I wait for the coffee to filter, I look at my digital screen and place my palm on it. I am identified by my palm print. Up on the screen comes an update on all my patients who have contacted the health system overnight. I log in to my online surgery and note that I have a video conference call with three patients, I email back to each of these with confirmation of their request.

Also on my screen is an alert regarding two potential changes to treatment. One of my patients has found a better treatment and contacted me to let me know. This will require me to change my practice and the nature of my support. The second alert is from Mrs Smith's automatic sensors which are built into her bathroom cabinet. The sensors have relayed that her blood sugar levels have been high each morning for the last six days; I make a note to contact her and see if there is a reason for this and if she needs some advice.

After I have dressed, I go out to the clinic and run my surgery, which is the usual mixture of one-to-one consultations and video link-ups. At lunchtime, I go online to take part in an international conference to update my understanding of development in my specialist field. I really enjoy the simulation, which enables me to start to practise a new technique for skin biopsy. The goggles I had to wear felt a bit strange at first. I note my interest in advancing in this area to the online local group, and a local mentor is highlighted. I expect him to get in touch with me later today.

A busy afternoon follows, but not so busy that I can't meet online with colleagues from across the locality to discuss new developments to facilities for health in the local community. I think the supermarkets' managers' idea for high-sugar goods to be placed on the top shelf is brilliant.

A final click and all my daily files are updated to the central system; I tag those patients who want an evening discussion; my colleague Jane will take over now. I chat to her briefly over the video phone link; she is based in the next town so we rarely meet yet I feel we work really well together. A good day.

This is a possible future scenario. In fact, all the technology referred to exists now and is in place in many parts of our health system but not necessarily joined up!

Reflective activity

Take a few moments to think about the sort of organisation you would like to work in, in the future.

- What would some of its key features be, particularly considering what you have read in the preceding chapters?
- What sort of structure and processes would need to be in place now to get things moving to make that future real?

Future organisations

Goold and Campbell (2002) carried out some research to consider what organisations of the future may look like. They saw several major themes driving current thinking, including:

- **Multidimensionality**. This involves moving away from a narrow focus on a single dimension, i.e., health services predominantly focused on illness, and being able to respond simultaneously to health across a broad range of dimensions, i.e., local, national, global, housing, environment.
- **Knowledge sharing**. The goal would be for every unit to seek out knowledge that is relevant to it from other units and to share its own knowledge with them. The organisation's structures and processes should be designed to facilitate this.
- **Desegregation**. As competition (expectations) intensifies, units and organisations need to concentrate on the activities that they do best. Taken to extremes, this can lead to the so-called 'virtual' organisation. Individual units have a high degree of autonomy, but cooperate together on a largely voluntary basis on those issues where there is a need to do so.
- **Freedom from hierarchy**. The focus should be on empowering front-line managers to take the initiative, and on enabling flatter, more responsive organisations. This requires the corporate centre to change its role, concentrating on resources and capability building.
- **Pursuing high performance**. There should be purposeful pursuit of high-performing strategies which always factor in the values-based activity as well as the financial imperative.

- **Renewal**. Owing to the pace of change, all organisations need to be able to constantly reinvent and renew themselves. This means being able to shift the focus of units flexibly as new opportunities/ expectations arise.

If you put these trends together, you will get a very different sort of organisation emerging, what some writers have called a **network organisation**. Networks in health systems score well as a possible design solution, as they meet the demands of some of the key challenges that we have identified in health throughout the earlier chapters.

Keywords

Network organisation
Is a multidimensional organisation consisting of many different units, each with its own focus

Networks are good at:

- Creating units that specialise in different aspects of health outcomes
- Encouraging cooperation between units by promoting interpersonal networking across unit boundaries
- Taking account of knowledge and competence by decentralising most responsibilities to individual focus units
- Reducing costs and fostering stronger commitment through self-management and clarity of purpose
- Reducing hierarchy and fostering more adaptable, flexible approaches to new opportunities

(adapted from Goold and Campbell, 2002)

Networks are becoming increasingly popular as a way of delivering complex clinical services over geographically spread populations. In the UK, networks have been actively used in the field of chronic disease management and have been particularly successful at improving services in cancer, coronary heart disease, and diabetes (see box below).

However, managing and leading in networks is a challenge; much depends on the motivation, flexibility and cooperativeness of you and your teams. Traditional behaviours, like sticking to the rules and regulations and being reluctant to collaborate with sister units, will guarantee that the network will fail.

Clinical networks

Clinical networks allow for a continuous working relationship between organisations and individuals to improve the treatment of patients who require care across a range of different institutions by, for example:

- making more efficient use of staff
- reducing professional and organisation boundaries
- sharing good practice
- putting the patient at the centre of care
- improving access to care

(NHS Service Development and Organisation, 2006, p. 2)

A recent report looking at network management highlighted some key points for developing successful networks (NHS Service Development and Organisation, 2006). Network coordination should:

- be proactive, and 'in control'
- have a clear statement of purpose and rules of engagement
- be inclusive to gain ownership
- actively engage respected professional leaders who will promote the network to peers
- develop strategies for network cohesion
- avoid network capture by dominant members
- also, large networks should be avoided as they become expensive to run and are too slow.

Clearly, networks are one sort of organisational form, but teams too are changing shape in response to the shifts in the context of care that we highlighted earlier. It is not uncommon for individual practitioners to be members of several teams simultaneously. Some of these teams may rarely meet: they are **virtual teams**.

Virtual teams

O─π Keywords

Virtual teams
Are teams of people who primarily interact electronically and who may occasionally meet face to face

> ### Reflective activity
>
> Think of an area of clinical practice in which you are involved. Now, start to think about the team.
> - Does the whole team meet up on a regular basis in the same space or are you a virtual team?
> - Do you think you need different skills to lead/manage a successful virtual team?

Virtual teams are certainly becoming more common; the reasons for this are many but, generally, centre on practicalities. For example, team members may not be physically co-located; travel to meetings is often expensive and, in terms of time, impractical; and team members may work different shifts. There is also the need to save time and, as we form alliances elsewhere to deliver health services, there may be additional reasons relating to the need to link with different countries and different time zones.

Fundamental processes that are well defined and agreed are as important for virtual teams as for traditional teams. These fundamentals include a shared vision, well-defined roles and responsibilities, project plans, meeting frameworks, and feedback on progress. Additionally, you will need to be able to understand and use information and communication technologies that support virtual teams.

Skills viewed as particularly important for the leadership and management of a virtual team are set out in the box below.

Virtual team leadership and management skills

- Ability to facilitate meetings (online, video, audio, face to face) including setting a positive tone electronically
- Ensuring that those team members who are not co-located are made to feel part of the team
- Technical proficiency with all communication tools in use by the team
- Spending significant time with team members not located with you
- Establishing a clear set of norms and protocols for behaviour
- Understanding and facilitating virtual-team development stages and dynamics
- Holding an initial face-to-face start-up meeting
- Using face-to-face meetings to resolve conflict and maintain team cohesiveness
- Remembering that reward and recognition for remote members may need to be more explicit
- Encouraging everyone to keep everyone else informed

Communities of practice

Although, as a leader/manager, you are likely to have professional accountability and responsibility for the outcomes of a range of formal networks associated with your organisation, it is worth noting that many of your ideas and much of your learning are products of less formal networks. These 'below the radar' networks have become the subject of a field of research into adult learning, because, when they exist, they can have many positive benefits (Wenger, 1999) (see Table 8.1).

Communities of practice can vary quite widely in their characteristics. Some exist for a long time, whilst others form for a short time, usually for a specific purpose. They are generally organic and self-organising, and, although organisations have tried to 'introduce' communities, these have often failed. Communities can, however, be encouraged to grow by the right organisational climate.

Communities differ from other teams in four key ways: they have voluntary membership; their focus is more general and fluid; they are not necessarily goal directed in their activities; and their existence is defined by their membership.

⚷ *Keywords*

Community of practice

Is a network of people who share a passion for something that they know how to do, and who interact regularly to learn how to do it better

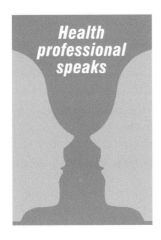

Specialist nurse

I am Janet; I work as a specialist nurse in the mental health field. About a year ago, I noticed that I had several teenage clients with a particular drug addiction. I felt very unprepared to support them, so I typed a query into the Internet. Before you knew it, I had found a small group that has set up an online discussion forum in this area. We meet occasionally (once every three months) as a UK group in a nearby town. It really has helped me to save time and give more effective support to my clients. We are also starting to lobby local politicians to make them more aware of what we believe to be a growing problem. We have attracted members from elsewhere in Europe, and they bring a very welcome range of alternative approaches to this difficult area. Although I will be leaving this role shortly, I will make sure that my colleague knows how to find this group: it's been a fantastic resource for me.

Table 8.1 Short- and long-term benefits to communities of practice

	Short-term value	Long-term value
Members	• Avoid reinventing the wheel • Help with challenges • Access to expertise • Increase confidence • Non-threatening forum to play with ideas	• Personal development • Professional development and enhanced identity • Network • Sharing • Generates new knowledge
Organisation	• Early-warning system for potential opportunities and threats • Time saving • Problem solving • Knowledge sharing • Reuse of resources	• Innovation • Retention of talent • Strategic learning • Creates a knowledge-sharing culture

(adapted from Wenger, 2004)

Supporting communities of practice

The successful fostering of communities of practice will require you (either as a member or a supporter) to get the balance right between giving them enough sponsorship to ensure their value, while at the same time not imposing too much structure and therefore risking losing the very relationships that underpin their effectiveness (Clemnon Rumizen, 2002). Particular roles that are important and should be explicitly supported are:

- coordinator (or leader) – organises and coordinates the community interactions and activities
- facilitator – facilitates the interactions within the community; this could be online or face to face

- knowledge manager – manages the explicit knowledge resources of the community, such as best practice guides, case studies, and locating and coordinating useful external resources.

Once the initial enthusiasm generated by setting up the community has passed, communities need active nourishing to prevent them from fading away. The ongoing success of a community relies on the constant encouragement of members' interest and involvement. A good coordinator will look for new challenges for the community, welcome and integrate new members, and move forward the body of knowledge in a wider range of opportunities.

Knowledge-based communities are already well established in many different types of organisations and have led to a much more detailed look at how knowledge itself is developed by individuals.

Over to you

Acknowledging that communities of practice affect performance is important in part because of their potential to overcome the inherent problems of slow-moving traditional hierarchy in a fast-moving virtual economy. Communities also appear to be an effective way for organisations to handle unstructured problems and to share knowledge outside of the traditional structural boundaries. In addition, the community concept is acknowledged to be a means of developing and maintaining long-term organisational memory. These outcomes are an important, yet often unrecognised, supplement to the value that individual members of a community obtain in the form of enriched learning and higher motivation to apply what they learn.

Lesser and Starck (2001, p. 837)

Consider the preceding quotation.

- Do you agree with the authors?
- Why do these communities present a problem to some organisations?
- Why do they make traditional managers so uncomfortable?

Keywords

Knowledge workers
Have high degrees of expertise, education, or experience, and the primary purpose of their jobs involves the creation, distribution, or application of knowledge

Knowledge workers

Another aspect of the changing nature of work and organisations is to think about how the needs of different types of workers can be met. An interesting perspective on this is put forward by Thomas Davenport (2005) who believes that it is critical that managers gain a much better understanding of just how to create the best environment for one of their key (and often expensive) assets: the **knowledge workers**. Health systems have a wide range of these individuals, for example physicians, scientists, and specialist practitioners.

So knowledge workers are those people whose jobs are particularly knowledge orientated; they enjoy their autonomy and are usually intelligent and highly committed to what they are doing.

Reflective activity

- Would you describe yourself as a knowledge worker?
- Do you think that knowledge workers as a group need special consideration?

Presumably, you have agreed that this group of workers has particular needs that may necessitate some changes in our approach. Davenport (2005) considers that managers will have to undergo some specific changes including moving:

- from overseeing work to doing it too (player/coaches)
- from organising hierarchies to organising communities
- from building manual skills to building knowledge skills
- from evaluating visible job performance to assessing invisible knowledge achievements
- from ignoring culture to building a knowledge-friendly culture
- from supporting bureaucracy to fending it off.

Knowledge management and knowledge transfer are exciting areas of development, and I am sure that we will be hearing a lot more about this field.

Pursuing high-performance strategies

There is, as we have noted, increasing emphasis on high-performance strategies in the workplace; for example, the Pursuing Perfection Programme in the NHS works to make promises to patients based upon their wants and needs.

A high-performance workplace (HPW) has been described as follows.

> A physical or virtual environment designed to enable workers to be as effective as possible in supporting business goals and promoting value. A HPW results from continually balancing investment in people, process, physical environment and technology, to measurably enhance the ability of workers to learn, discover, innovate, team and lead, and to achieve efficiency and financial benefit.
>
> Gartner (2005)

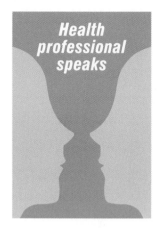

A nurse manager

What a day! What is it about the Larch unit; why do they have so many problems? I just don't get it. Ash ward is right next door: same layout, same client group, similar staffing, similar budget and nothing like the problems; they just seem to quietly get on. How can one unit get it so right and the other get it so wrong? I know which one I would want my mum to go to if she needed care.

Reflective activity

If you were asked to recommend a good unit, would you recommend your own?

In some ways, looking for the answer as to why some organisations and teams are so good and some are so bad can feel like an impossible quest, like looking for buried treasure. However, a recent large-scale piece of research by Bevan *et* al. (2005), published by the Work Foundation, sought to explain why the UK has simultaneously produced some of the most innovative and successful companies in the world, and some of its least inspiring and most unambitious. The results of this research programme provide us with some surprising answers.

Cracking the performance code

Structures

The exact structure and shape deployed seems to make little difference to high performing organisations. Though a topic beloved by bosses and human resource teams in slow-moving bureaucracies, the exact organisational shape seems to matter little for the more successful firms. Whilst there were some general themes about how high-performing companies organise themselves to manufacture their product or deliver their services, it was significant that no single organisational design seemed to emerge. This aspect of organisational life did not seem to be that important.

Some of the consistent features tended to be aspects like flatter structures and some form of matrix working but, beyond this, organisation design appeared to be more a function of size, geography and history.

It seems fair to conclude that, for high-performing companies, structure is more likely to be an enabler than a driver of success and that form is more likely to follow 'function'.

Processes

The top firms were also characterised by the apparent simplicity of their processes (although 'simple' should not be confused with 'simplistic'). Such minimalist organisational processes are driven by a general philosophy that 'less is more' and by strong communications up, down and across the organisation.

'Meetings' were often referred to as an unnecessary hindrance and talk of steering committees and work groups was conspicuous by its absence. The outcome, universally, was that decisions happen faster this way and that, even if they turn out not to be the right ones, adjusting course and actions afterwards can happen just as quickly too. Similarly, performance management was kept simple.

Communication

High performance means good communication between peers and an apparent willingness for managers to share openly all relevant information both to individuals and representative staff bodies such as Trades Unions and Works Councils. Communication and the steady flow of information not only up and down, but also across the organisation, were typically seen as a strength by all levels of staff.

'Knowledge is power' was not in evidence but 'knowledge sharing' was very much seen as a core organisational objective especially to those acting at the customer interface.

Leadership

Openness, visibility and accessibility were characteristics of the prevailing leadership and management style in high-performing business. More apparent was a general lack of hierarchy accompanied by a strong focus to give people access to the resources, information and technology they needed to get the job done effectively. As reflected in culture, these organisations had equal measures of task and people-orientation.

Leaders in these firms appear to set high standards and expectations of everyone around them but, at the same time, are aware of their position as role models. However the stewardship model of leadership emerging is light years away from the visionary leadership model beloved by the business press.

Culture and employee relations

In the high-performing firms there were some clear cultural norms. First there was a distrust of the status quo. These organisations also valued quality over quantity, an external as well as internal focus and had a sense of pride about their 'reason to be'. Managers seemed to have a positive self-image, be concerned about their own development and expect others to think the same way too. These behavioural norms clearly underpin cultural manifestations of leadership style and internal communication.

A long-term orientation around the needs of the customer was similarly evident. Elsewhere, knowing the business, pursuing excellence and subordinating processes and structure to outcomes and delivery were evidence of a strong achievement orientation. People had some real influence over what goes on in their work unit. Allowing workers as much control as possible over when, where and how the job is done is a key feature of the high performing firms we studied.

This restless curiosity and achievement focus seems to show through also in the employee relations philosophy of many of the top firms. Support, loyalty and long service aligned to the broader organisational strategies were much in evidence. A set of positive employee outcomes around pride, engagement and motivation seemed more associated with a challenging, open and dynamic working environment than merely with a culture of friendliness and strong interpersonal relationships. Trust and respect were products of solidarity rather than simple sociability.

(Bevan *et al.*, 2005)

These key behaviours offer a helpful template for reflecting on our own organisation and key behaviours within it. It is also possible to see that many of the themes that we have explored throughout the book to date are encapsulated in the findings.

Recognising myths and fads

What the findings of Bevan *et al.* (2005) also challenge is the celebrity culture which has built up around some of our leaders and managers. They underline the value of a less visible form of leadership, what Badarocco (2003) terms 'quiet leadership'. Badarocco (2003) believes that our current preoccupation with leadership and management heroes (gurus) gives us a distorted view of the organisation and has three serious drawbacks.

- It encourages us to think of the organisation as a pyramid with stars at the top. (You have probably heard people say, 'Look out for the rising stars'.) But what does that mean for everyone else?
- It portrays great leaders as confronting great challenges: but what if the real problems are smaller and messier and the answer is less straightforward?
- It offers little help to people dealing with the uncertainties of our real world, which is different and unique in comparison with what has gone before.

Reflective activity

Think of someone whom you greatly admire but who is not famous.

- How do they influence? Is it in small ways, which seem to add up, or is it in grand gestures?
- Do you encourage and recognise the small achievements of patients, co-workers, and family?

A mosquito is a good example of how a small thing can have a system-wide impact!

Characteristics of quiet leaders

Badarocco (2003) became so interested in this notion of quiet leaders, that he carried out some research to look at how people in the middle of organisations successfully addressed everyday issues. He came up with some interesting findings. The people he studied were very pragmatic. They worked quietly behind the scenes with a clear goal of addressing serious problems and living by their values. They did not assume that 'the right answer' was obvious. Heroism, in their view, was a last resort, not a first choice. As Badarocco (2003) notes:

> in other words, preparation, caution, care and attention to detail are usually the best approach to important and demanding challenges.
>
> Badarocco (2003, p. 3)

The research suggests six basic guidelines for successful quiet leadership (see box).

Successful quiet leadership

- Quiet leaders see the world as a kaleidoscope rather than a well-planned map
- Quiet leaders reject cynicism as too narrow a view
- Quiet leaders are tenacious; they have a constancy of purpose
- Quiet leaders buy time – they respond rather than react
- Quiet leaders use the time they buy to really understand the complexity of the issue facing them
- Quiet leaders look for compromises; they try and generate wiggle room in tight situations

---

Middle managers

Illuminating the often invisible but nonetheless effective leaders and managers of an organisation is clearly a critical challenge. As organisations look to the future and change their shapes, they can run the risk of designing out the very features that help make them work. A good example of this is the role of middle managers. This level of management is frequently the source of much criticism; middle managers are often vulnerable to redundancy and the target of political pressure, yet recent research carried out in Canada points to the crucial role that middle managers play in implementing change (Golden Biddle *et al.*, 2003). Their key asset is that they know how to get things done because they are very knowledgeable about the organisation. Regardless of the health care setting, the middle managers studied faced three common challenges:

- **Clarifying the reallocation of tasks**. During change, middle managers help to sort out the 'Who does what?' question that new roles/practices create.
- **Managing altered working relationships within the team**. The managers help staff to answer the question 'Where do I fit in?'

- **Continuing to manage the team in an evolving situation**. Effective managers work to develop overall goals in answer to the 'What happens next?' question.

The research goes on to make several suggestions as to how organisations can more purposefully tap into the capability of their middle managers.

- Look closely at how the organisation supports the important relationship the middle managers have with their front-line staff.
- Recognise the knowledge that these managers have as a valuable resource and use it to inform decision making.
- Find ways to minimise the constraining factors above and below them in the organisation.
- Acknowledge and reward the work of middle managers.

Reflective activity

Think of the relationship that you have with managers around you at work. Look at the suggestions listed in the previous paragraph.

- Do you think that by taking up some of these suggestions you could enhance your relationships?
- Do you ever hear people referring to managers as 'them' and unit team members as 'us'? If so, would you now challenge this language?

⚷ Keywords

Fad

Is a fashion that is taken up with great enthusiasm for a brief period of time

Changing focus

Perhaps, as we look to challenge some of the **fads** and myths around us, it is also important to be aware that some of the skills that we say we will need in the future can also have a negative effect if over-pursued. For example, too intense a focus on achievement, which is often associated with command and control behaviours, can demolish trust and morale.

In many organisations, the corporate (senior-level) leaders are not having a good time. Quality scandals, large pay increases and more focused public scrutiny have made their world a much less comfortable place. At the same time, many leaders, particularly of large public sector organisations, are being pressed to answer deeper and more complex questions than ever before. Instead of simply focusing on questions of performance, activity and costs, leaders are now being challenged to respond to questions of meaning and purpose (Broome and Hughes, 2004). For example, just because we can provide a particular service should we? Should we carry out genetic screening for gender? Should we keep people alive on life support as a right? Should we offer a bathing service to elderly people?

As we noted earlier, it is the relationship between people that results in action. Followers need leaders who can let them know that what they do is important, and how it makes a difference (Department of Trade and Industry, 2004), even if that is a difficult call to make at times.

This shift in the focus of leadership and management has led to a significant increase in development opportunities and a growing recognition of the importance of considering the emotional and ethical aspects of leadership and management activities. Such topics as genuineness, authenticity, credibility and trustworthiness are actively explored in relation to the needs of organisations, teams and individuals for the future. The next section starts with examples of three such approaches: servant leadership, authentic leadership, and emotional intelligence.

Approaches to leadership

Keywords

Servant leadership

Is a practical philosophy, which supports people who choose to serve first and then lead as a way of expanding service to individuals and institutions

Servant leadership

Servant leadership encourages collaboration, trust, foresight, listening, and the ethical use of power and empowerment.

Robert Greenleaf (2002) distinguishes the servant leader as an individual who chooses to serve first and then become a leader, rather than the converse.

Keywords

Authentic leadership

Is an approach that sees leadership as authentic self-expression that creates value

Authentic leadership

Kevin Cashman (2000) sees the foundation of leadership as being authenticity. He suggests that there are five touchstones that are crucial to build the interpersonal bridge essential for **authentic leadership**:

- know yourself authentically – practise being what you wish others to become
- listen authentically – centred in the principle of reciprocity
- express authentically – congruence between who we are and what we do
- appreciate authentically
- serve authentically – move from control to serving.

Emotional intelligence

Supporters of the concept of emotional intelligence (EI) argue that conventional intelligence is too narrow and that there are wider areas of emotional intelligence that contribute to how successful we are.

Daniel Goleman (1995) identified five domains of EI:

- knowing your emotions
- managing your emotions

- motivating yourself
- recognising and understanding other people's emotions
- managing relationships.

Goleman (1995) argues that, by developing our EI in these areas, we can become more productive and successful at what we do and help others to achieve more too.

All the models presented in this section have their critics as well as their fans. However, they serve to underline a broader trend, which is that we should be able to articulate a sound framework of values as part of our approach to leading and managing for the future.

In a survey of corporate leadership, *The Economist* listed a 10-point checklist of qualities necessary for a good 'boss' in the future. Do you think that these could apply to your sector?

10 top qualities

1. A sound ethical compass – good people like to work for organisations whose values they trust

2. The ability to make difficult decisions – many judgements are made on incomplete information, and this will mean mistakes, risk and upset, but a decision is better than no decision

3. Clarity and focus – extracting the crucial point from complexity is essential for achieving an effective strategy; so too, is the ability to screen out noise and focus on what really matters

4. Ambition – the best leaders want to create something that outlasts them

5. Effective communication skills – presenting a vision clearly requires a persuasive leader who can inspire trust and convey authenticity

6. The ability to judge people – judging who will work best and where is a key task, needing experience and intuition

7. A knack for developing talent – people learn a lot from a good mentor; all leaders need to be teachers

8. Emotional self-confidence – self-confidence enables you to admit your limitations and ask help from colleagues without losing their respect

9. Adaptability – the ability to reframe and reshape problems increases the chances of a flexible response

10. Charm – few get to the top without it

(adapted from A Survey of Corporate Leadership, *The Economist*, 2003)

Up until now, this chapter, like the preceding ones, has tried to set out a variety of possibilities. These possibilities relate to how your understanding of the key dimensions of leadership and management can begin to help you to influence the future that you would wish to see for yourself and for the people whom you seek to serve. We have actively sought to encourage you to start to visualise what organisations may look like in the future and to think. However, by definition, the future is unknown, and we all have to live in the now. So what are you going to do now to create the future?

Developing your future dimensions

The final challenge of this book is to help you to take personal ownership of your leadership and management development and translate it into real changes with a *personal vision* for your development.

This vision is your vision: what you are going to change; what you are going to do differently with your team, friends and family in order to be more effective. It involves being self-aware and achieving the right balance for you.

Over to you

On a large sheet of paper, write or draw your responses to the following questions; try to avoid writing your answers in a list. If you see connections between your ideas, then show the link by, for example, using arrows or colour.

- What would you like to achieve?
- What kind of a leader would you wish people to describe you as?
- Do you have a belief or principle that you hold true to whatever the context?
- How would you describe yourself?
- What would you wish to be remembered for?
- What could you teach others to do?
- What would you like to do most often?
- What new skills would you like to develop?
- Are you willing to make sacrifices to achieve your personal vision?

Stand back from your sheet and see if you can come up with two statements that complete the following two sentences.

1. In two years, I will be . . .
2. You will know that I am effective in this because you will see me . . .

Personal development plan

Having identified where you expect to be and what you will be doing, the next step is to think systematically about those things that you will need in place in order to reach your goal.

Although there will be formal learning opportunities that would help, such as taking additional qualifications, remember that non-course-based learning can be equally (if not more) important. Consider activities such as job shadowing, getting a mentor, being coached. But perhaps the biggest challenge of all in relation to adopting new behaviours is to confront some of your existing ways of thinking and assumptions about yourself and others.

Certain assumptions can be made about the process of growth:

- You can change your life. Events of the past have an influence and are important but they do not control your future.
- You know more than you think you do, and you probably underestimate your own abilities.
- Building a different world may require change; some of the change may be hard, but equally some will be simple and easy.
- Building a more positive world should be fun.
- As you change your life, you will change the life of others around you.
- It is important for you to be sure you want what you think you want (adapted from Management Research Group, 2006).

Reflective activity

Success is whatever you say it is, not a goal defined by your family, friends, work colleagues or even the media. If you measure success only in objectives reached, money earned and publications cited, then you may find yourself saying, 'Is that all there is?' Think about success as coming in other guises. Find a quiet spot and consider the following:

- What is your definition of success? Do you consider yourself successful? Would others?
- Whose ideas about success have most influenced you? Would this need to change if you are to be successful on your own terms?
- Who are your models of success? What is it you admire about them? Can you find these qualities in yourself?

In order to give yourself the best chance of completing the change process, you will need to define your goals. They should be very concrete and real for you. Consider the following questions as you choose your goal:

- Can you state the goal in specific terms? 'I will . . . '
- Is the goal realistic for you to achieve?
- Can you achieve it in a set time frame?
- Do you have a strong commitment to this goal?

You may find it helpful to use the five steps shown in the following box as a template for an action plan.

Action plan

1. Summarise your goal
2. Evaluate and describe those resources which could help you reach this goal (people, things, institutions)
3. What could get in the way of your achieving your goal? How will you overcome these difficulties?
4. Describe your actions and assign a completion/review date
5. To whom will you communicate the goal? Why and how?

Remember that leadership and management is a practical art which is learnt by experience; we are all both teachers and learners.

Finally, reflect once again on the 3-dimensional approach to leadership and management (see figure below).

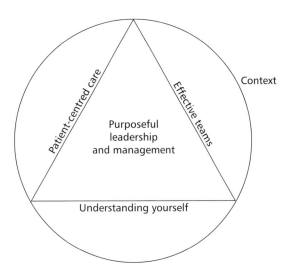

A 3-dimensional approach to leadership and management

Remember the exercise that we carried out (see Chapter 1, pp. 17–19). Are there any aspects of your development plan that you would wish to add to in the light of your reflections?

Conclusion

As the proceeding chapters have shown, several trends will play a major role in our future understanding and development of leadership and management skills. These trends represent the critical role played by changing contexts in health systems.

- Competence in leadership and management skills will continue to matter, but how they are evaluated will change as accountabilities broaden.
- Patient-led services will require that leaders/managers deal with a broader range of stakeholders in a global context.
- Owing to technology's growing role, there will continue to be radical changes in organisational life, and leaders and managers will need to anticipate and respond to these.
- There will be increasing emphasis on the integrity and character of leaders and managers.

The world of contemporary organisations is complex, filled with challenges and opportunities. In order to grow and develop, organisations, whatever their shape, need a fully engaged workforce. All members of the health system are being asked to evaluate services in their areas and offer better ways of doing things, and each person has the power to create new visions and new realities. The organisation needs to generate the right culture to ensure the participation of all. We are all responsible for contributing to this culture but doing so requires us to challenge ourselves and others to expand their efforts, break down barriers to achievement, and exceed expectations. We need to be purposeful in our leadership and management endeavours.

RRRRRRapid recap

Check your progress so far by working through each of the following questions:

1. List four advantages to an organisation of having communities of practice.
2. Identify six key qualities for a future 'boss'.
3. What would be the key aspects of culture that would need to be in place to foster a high-performance workplace?

If you have difficulty with more than one of the questions, read through the section again to refresh your understanding before moving on.

References

Badarocco, J.L. (2003) A Lesson for the Times: Learning from Quiet Leaders. *Ivey Business Journal* (Jan.–Feb.): 1–6.

Bevan, S. *et al.* (2005) *Cracking the Performance Code: How Firms Succeed*. The Work Foundation, London.

Broome, G. and Hughes, R.L. (2004) Leadership Development: Past, Present and Future. *Human Resource Planning*, **27**(1): 24–32.

Cashman, K. (2000) *Leadership from the Inside Out*. Executive Excellence, Provo, UT.

Clemnon Rumizen, M. (2002) *The Complete Idiot's Guide to Knowledge Management*. Civil Publishing Enterprises, Madison.

Davenport, T.H. (2005) *Thinking for a Living*. Harvard Business School Press, Boston.

Department of Trade and Industry (2004) *Inspired Leadership: Insights into People who Inspire Exceptional Performance*, www.dti.gov.uk.

Gartner Inc. (2005) *The High Performance Workplace Defined*, www.gartner.com.

Golden Biddle, H., Reay, T. and Thomson, D. (2003) Implementing Change: The Crucial Role of Middle Managers. *Health Organisation Studies* (Nov.): 1–3. www.bus.ualberta.ca/hos.

Goleman, D. (1995) *Emotional Intelligence*. Bantam, New York.

Goold, M. and Campbell, A., (2002) *Designing Effective Organisations: How to Create Structured Networks*. Wiley, Chichester.

Greenleaf, R. (2002) *Servant Leadership: A Journey into the Nature of Legitimate Power and Greatness*. Paulist Press, Ramsey, NJ.

Lesser, E.L. and Starck, J. (2001) Communities of Practice and Organisational Performance. *IBM Systems Journal*, **40**(4): 831–841.

Management Research Group (2006) *Personal Directions*. www.mrg.com.

NHS Service Development and Organisation (2006) *Key Lessons for Network Management in Healthcare*. NHS SDO, London.

The Economist (2003). A Survey of Corporate Leadership (25 Oct.): 3–26. Economist.com/surveys.

Wenger, E., (1999) *Communities of Practice: Learning Meanings and Identity*. Cambridge University Press, Cambridge.

Wenger, E. (2004) *Cultivating Communities of Practice*. www.ewenger.com/theory.

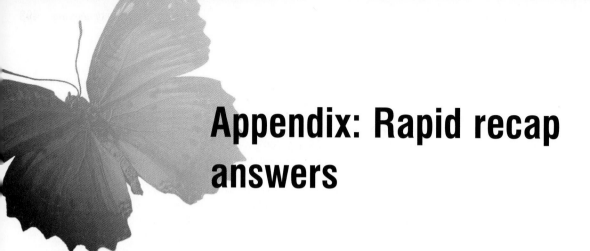

Appendix: Rapid recap answers

Chapter One

1. **List six major trends that are currently actively influencing the development of health systems.**

   Some of the major trends that are currently active in influencing the development of health systems are changes in the:
   - health needs profile, e.g. changes in the age of the population, the prevalence of different illnesses and epidemics
   - health systems, e.g. funding for health, technology, and consumer expectations
   - context, e.g. health service reform, workforce changes and education, worldwide sharing of information
   - numbers, e.g. skills shortages and skill mix, over-supply, generational balance
   - distribution, e.g. primary/secondary, international migration
   - workforce conditions, pay and rewards, lifelong learning, workplace safety.

2. **Describe two differences between a leader and a manager.**

   Differences between a leader and manager are that:
   - a **leader** challenges, develops a long-term focus, is visionary, is people focused, asks what and why, mentors, is innovative, and develops trust, whereas
   - a **manager** plans, coordinates, controls, directs, asks how and why, is task focused, organises, is present orientated, focuses on the short term, and is reactive.

3. **Describe four activities that would support the adoption of a new idea.**

   Activities that would support the adoption of a new idea are:

   - find sound innovations
   - find and support innovators
   - invest in early adopters
   - make early adopter activity observable
   - trust and enable reinvention
   - create slack for change
   - lead by example.

4. **What would be four key features of a culture that fostered improvements in care?**

   Key features of a culture that fostered improvements in care are:
   - Achievement focus – focus on key strategic tasks and initiatives that everyone in the organisation must be aware of and subscribe to.
   - Overcome fear of failure – upbringing and culture can make us risk adverse. As leaders we need to encourage experimentation and risk taking.
   - Access your inner self – this urges us to use intuition and experience to spot ideas, trends and patterns, which helps us make sense of things more quickly.
   - Simple questions, simple answers – as we can so easily become overloaded with information, simple, clear and concise communication about the direction and goals of the organisation is essential.
   - Energy and fun – an energised team is a creative and effective force.

5. **List the four elements of the McNichol and Hamer 3-dimensional model of leadership and management.**

   The four elements of the McNichol and Hamer 3-dimensional model of leadership and management are:
   - purposeful leadership and management

- patient-centred care
- effective teamworking
- understanding yourself.

Chapter Two

1. **Describe the difference between position power and personal power.**

   Position power is associated with the position that you hold and not with you as a person; it comprises connection, legitimate, coercive and reward facets of power. In contrast, personal power is the power that you have as an individual, irrespective of your job title. Personal power is described in terms of expert, information and referent power.

2. **Name five mental locks that people use that inhibit their creative ability.**

   Possible mental locks include:
   - the right answer
   - be practical
   - don't be foolish
   - that's not logical
   - we don't have time
   - to err is wrong
   - follow the rules
   - that's not my area
   - I'm not creative.

   There may well be some others that you could include that are particularly pertinent to you.

3. **How could you use the Whole Brain Model to help you at work?**

   You can use the model in a number of ways, including:
   - to improve communication through a greater appreciation of different preferences and of how these influence how people talk and act
   - team building, by understanding the impact of preferences or avoidances in relation to the four quadrants of the model
   - preparing effective presentations, by using the model as a checklist to see that you have addressed all four quadrants within your presentation.

4. **Why might 'learner' questions enable you to move a situation forward further than if you were using 'judger' questions?**

   Learner path questions begin from the perspective of wanting to understand a situation or circumstance so that you as an individual are able to move forward in your thinking and approach in order to make positive progress. The method is very much underpinned by a solution-focused and learning philosophy, which helps to build confidence, encourages personal responsibility and supports positive working relationships. In contrast, judger path questions tend to focus on *who* or *what* went wrong in order to find the 'cause' of the problem and name it. Whilst it is important to identify specific problems and address them, very often judger path questions take you down a road of blame, either of others or of yourself. The consequences can then be a fear of failure, loss of confidence to try new things and a 'half-empty glass' perspective on the world.

5. **Identify the four key words of the Fish philosophy and describe how you could make them relevant to your world.**

   The four key words of the Fish Philosophy are:
   - play
   - make their day
   - be there
   - choose your attitude.

   In your description of how the key words could be relevant to your world, try to go beyond work and consider your life as a whole.

6. **Identify five developmental activities that you could include in a personal development plan.**

   The following are all possible developmental options:
   - job rotation
   - extend your scope of practice
   - become a mentor for someone else
   - read books/journals
   - seek feedback
   - visit other comparable work-places
   - work shadowing
   - training in specific skills
   - form/join an action learning set
   - visit relevant websites
   - keep a learning diary/log
   - attend special-interest meetings

- secondments
- find an appropriate mentor
- tap into new networks
- undertake some research
- volunteer for a working or project group.

Chapter Three

1. **What is the difference between a 'reaction' and a 'response'?**

   A reaction is an automatic thought, behaviour or action with no real thought behind it. This is fine in life-threatening situations that require you to act on instinct but is not appropriate for the majority of management-related decisions that a health care professional needs to take.

   In contrast, making a response means that you stopped, pressed the PAUSE button, thought about your options and chose one of them. The difference is that you are more in control of yourself and therefore have more choice about how to deal with the situation.

2. **Briefly define the concepts of 'care-taker' and 'rescuer'.**

   A 'care-taker' is someone who does things for other people that those people are quite capable of doing themselves. You may behave like this for any number of reasons, such as a desire to help others out or because you want to be liked. However, the core component is that you have chosen to take on the role, generally because it fulfils a need in you.

   A 'rescuer' is someone who bails people out of difficult situations as opposed to holding on to the safety line and ensuring that they stay afloat whilst they work their way to safety. Again, it is likely that you voluntarily take on this role: perhaps you are uncomfortable seeing people in difficulty or you accept it when someone shouts 'help'; or it maybe that, for you, it is quicker or easier than helping others to stay afloat and work their way through the situation.

3. **What type of time-management activities could be classed as 'important:not urgent'?**

   The type of management activities that are 'important:not urgent' include:

   - practice and service development initiatives
   - patient-focused activities
   - activity concerned with preventing future crises

- relationship-building initiatives – in team and with wider partners
- innovative thinking and idea development
- ensuring that important things become routine, e.g. good record keeping, standards of care.

4. **What is the value of working within your circle of influence as opposed to your circle of concern?**

   The value of working within your circle of influence is that you use your time and energy effectively to focus your energies proactively on things that you can influence. This is generally more motivating and rewarding than operating within your circle of concern, where you have less opportunity to influence and are more likely to slide into 'complaining' behaviour.

5. **What are the six points of Maxwell's A's and E's quality framework?**

   The six points are:

   - accessibility of the service by all who need it
   - acceptability of the service to society, its users and stakeholders
   - appropriateness or relevance of the service to the community
   - effectiveness of the service for individuals
   - equity and fairness of the service
   - efficiency and economy of the service.

Chapter Four

1. **List three characteristics of a team.**

   A team:

   - shares objectives
   - has the necessary authority, autonomy and resources to achieve these objectives
   - has to work closely and interdependently to achieve these objectives
   - has well-defined and unique roles
   - is recognised as a team
   - includes no fewer than 3 and no more than 15 members.

2. **Identify and describe four types of groups or teams.**

   Types of groups or teams include:

   - **Working group**: members interact primarily to share information and views, coordinate practices, etc. There is little shared responsibility – the emphasis is on individual responsibility, and there is no significant need or opportunity requiring it to become a team

- **Pseudo-team**: not really focused on communal responsibility and coordination and is not trying to achieve it. Less impact than working groups because interactions detract from members' individual performance without delivering any joint benefits

- **Potential team**: trying to improve performance impact, but lacks clarity about shared goals and individual accountability to the team and working practices

- **Real team**: a small group of people with complementary skills, who are equally committed to a common purpose, goal and working approach, for which they hold themselves mutually accountable

- **High-performance team**: a group that meets all the conditions of real teams and has members who are deeply committed to each other's personal growth and success (Katzenback and Smith, 1993, p. 91)

- **Virtual teams**: 'virtual' implies that the common workplace is via technology, meaning that team members may be in the same (co-located) or different (distributed) locations so that their communication and information sharing may be synchronous (at the same time) or asynchronous (in different time zones). The combination of advances in communication and increasing globalisation and competition means that individuals anywhere in the world can interact on the move and share information (Buchanan and Huczynski, 2004, p. 309)

- **Self-directed teams**: teams that share the leading rather than having one single leader; the person best suited to the task takes the lead. The evaluation of performance and achievement of goals is by mutual accountability. In discussion about the training of marines, Katzenbach and Santamaria describe how the groups are highly cohesive and are able to learn when to use real team and single-leader team to best advantage (Buchanan and Huczynski, 2004, p. 308).

3. **List the five leadership strategies of the CLIMB model.**

The five leadership strategies associated with the CLIMB model are:

Create a compelling future

Let the customer drive the organisation

Involve every mind

Manage work horizontally

Build personal credibility.

4. **What are the competencies displayed by successful teams?**

Successful teams display the following competencies:

1. Patient and/or carer focus: establish and maintain effective relationships with patient and/or carers

1a Establish and maintain effective two-way relationships with patients

1b Enable patient and/or carers to make informed decisions

1c Contribute to and support the decision-making process

2. Team focus: establish and maintain effective team delivery

2a Understand the range of roles within service-delivery team and how their strengths and limitations can contribute to effective patient care

2b Assume service team leadership in decision making

2c Contribute to the development of an effective team ethos and vision

3. Interpersonal understanding and impact: identify and understand others' needs and concerns and modify own response to build credibility, mutual respect and trust

3a Establish and maintain effective relationships with team members

3b Maintain personal stability when under pressure

4 Quality assurance: contribute to the process of continuous improvement in patient and/or carers' care

4a Commitment to improve own performance in order to improve the delivery of patient care

4b Review team performance in order to improve the delivery of patient care.

5. **What are the behaviours that you should exhibit when your team is less successful?**

When your team is less successful, you should:

- Keep reminding yourself of the vision/purpose.
- Write down reasons that you took the job/profession, renewing your passion.

- Seek to understand, check out assumptions.
- Seek out supervision or mentoring.
- Lead by example, model good time management and professional appearance.
- Reinforce all positives, possibilities, opportunities and potential.
- Don't reciprocate practices that you want to end.

Chapter Five

1. How can effectiveness be defined?

Effectiveness can be defined as:

- safety
- clinical and cost effectiveness
- governance
- patient focus
- accessible and responsive care
- care environment and amenities
- public health (Standards for Better Health, 2006).

2. What are the key areas that everyone is accountable for delivering to ensure effectiveness in health care?

The key areas that everyone is accountable for delivering to ensure effectiveness in health care are:

- safety
- clinical and cost effectiveness
- governance
- patient focus
- accessible and responsive care
- care environment and amenities
- public health.

3. What is the purpose of a SMART objective and what does the acronym stand for?

SMART is a specific objective that is set out so that it is clear who is doing what and by when. SMART is an acronym:

Specific

Measurable

Achievable

Realistic

Timebound.

4. Name and describe four of the roles identified by Belbin that people adopt when working in teams.

The roles identified by Belbin that people adopt when working in teams are:

- Plant – creates imaginative ideas, proposes novel solutions to difficult problems, prefers to work alone, sensitive to praise and criticism
- Resource-investigator – good communicator, enthusiastic, extrovert, likes networking, good at negotiation, easily bored
- Coordinator – good chairperson, delegates well, clarifies and promotes decision making; good at recognising an individual's abilities and getting them involved; keeps the group on track towards the objective
- Shaper – highly motivated, thrives on pressure, challenging, needs to achieve; can appear pushy and aggressive
- Monitor-evaluator – steady, not displaying excesses of emotion, strategic and serious; sees the options and critically judges slowly but accurately
- Teamworker – diplomatic and cooperative; provides support for others in the team; avoids conflict and allows others to contribute to the task
- Implementer – efficient, practical, reliable; likes routine and being systematic
- Completer – conscientious, gives attention to detail, anxious; relies on themselves and delivers on time with high standards
- Specialist – has specific technical skill, focused, dedicated; more interested in their professional standards than in the team's work and its members.

5. How can you encourage an appropriate feedback culture in your team?

You can encourage an appropriate feedback culture in your team by:

- seeking feedback for yourself
- being open and responsive to feedback
- fostering open and honest discussion
- building relationships
- understanding what each other needs
- giving time for feedback.

6. **Identify five features of a solution-focused approach.**

Five features of a solution-focused approach are:

- acknowledge the problem – how is it a problem to you?
- define how you would like the future to be
- find out what helps to make progress towards this future
- do more of what works
- if something does not work, stop and do something else.

Chapter Six

1. **Provide a working definition of the term 'patient-centred care'.**

At the most basic level, patient-centred care can be defined as care that considers the values, preferences and needs of individual patients. At a more collective level, it means thinking about how patients or other members of the public can be involved in strategic planning and service development.

2. **Identify at least four important events or changes that have occurred since the beginnings of the NHS that have contributed to current reforms.**

Important events or changes that have occurred since the beginnings of the NHS that have contributed to current reforms are:

- 1960s – a series of reports detailing poor quality care for the elderly and mentally ill
- 1974 – the introduction of Community Health Councils
- 1979 – the election of a government committed to radical reform
- 1983 –the Griffiths Report and the introduction of general management and the concept of the patient as a consumer
- 1991 – the Allitt Inquiry
- 2001 – the Bristol Inquiry Report
- 2004 – the Shipman Inquiry.

3. **What is the main role of the government in patient-led services?**

The main role of government in patient-led services is to:

- turn public values into public policy

- engage the public, seek their opinions and use them to inform policy
- plan for the future in consultation with the public
- make information more readily available.

4. **Describe at least one action that health care provider organisations or senior managers can take to move services toward patient-centred provision.**

To move services towards patient-centred provision, health care provider organisations or senior managers can:

- honour service standards, e.g. waiting times
- ensure that services will be coordinated and convenient for the patient
- ensure that staff are pleasant and knowledgeable and assist patients when needed.

5. **Define 'empathy' and its role in patient-centred leadership.**

Empathy is the ability to share and understand the feelings of another. It is an important facet of patient-centred leadership. Empathy allows you to concentrate on the other person and incorporates notions of respect and effective communication. Empathy is both an emotional quality and a behaviour. When interacting with patients, you need to demonstrate active empathetic listening. Empathetic listening means to listen not only for the facts, but also for the emotional impact of the situation. Facts and emotions together create a rich picture of the patient experience as a whole. A rich picture is a very useful tool for exercising patient-centred leadership.

6. **What is meant by the term a 'patient-led NHS'?**

A patient-led NHS involves more than service development and choice; it is about responding to and being led by the needs and wishes of patients. (Department of Health, 2005).

Chapter Seven

1. **Describe the difference between patient-centred management and managing the patient.**

Differences are that when:

- **managing the patient**, services are designed by professionals and are available in business hours; decisions are made by professionals; patients are passed from service to service, professional to professional; it is assumed that the professional knows best and gives advice, whereas

- **in patient-centred management,** services are designed by patients and are available at all hours; decisions are made by patients; services are moved closer to the patients or coordinated to create a 'one-stop' service whenever possible; it is assumed that the patient knows best; information is given and discussed.

Patient-centred management is a process of designing and delivering services that accommodate the needs, beliefs and preferences of each individual with a view to creating a good experience as judged by that individual. The most important principle underpinning patient-centred service design and delivery is how it will meet the needs of the patients using the service. In contrast, managing the patient generally means fitting the patient into a health care system that has traditionally been designed around health care staff and existing health care structures.

2. **Describe five things that could turn a satisfactory event into a satisfying experience.**

Instances where a satisfactory event could turn into a satisfying experience are:

- fast access to reliable health care
- effective treatment delivered by trusted professionals
- involvement in decisions and respect for preferences
- clear, comprehensive information and support for self-care
- attention to physical and environmental needs
- emotional support, empathy and respect
- involvement of, and support for, family and carers
- continuity of care and smooth transitions.

3. **What actions can be taken to create a more equal perception of power between health care providers and patients?**

To create a more equal perception of power between health care providers and patients:

- Visit your belief system regarding your role in caring for patients. Do you believe that the patient is your equal? The patient is capable, intelligent and experienced and should be fully involved in every aspect of their care. We share

responsibilities: I am responsible for sharing my expertise and the patient is responsible for weighing the information, and choosing the course of action best for them.

- Actively facilitate the principle of patient empowerment. This means building the knowledge and confidence of individuals to enable them to participate effectively, to the extent that they wish, in their own care.
- Remember that empowerment can extend to enabling patients or members of the public to participate in the planning, evaluation and design of health services for other people.
- Learn actively from complaints and compliments.

4. **Identify three conversational ways of moving a long-standing, unequal relationship between nurse and patient to one where the relationship is more equal and patient centred.**

To begin to create a more equal, patient-centred relationship, you could:

- Tell the patient how you are feeling about the situation – 'Mrs H, I have been seeing you for a year now, and I now feel that you are very capable of managing your diabetes care, and I think it is appropriate that my visits stop. I would be sad about that because I really enjoy visiting you. I am concerned that we seem to be stuck, with neither of us moving on in the way we should.'
- Tell the patient what you want – 'Mrs H, I want to work out a way for my visits to decrease and eventually stop, in a way that doesn't upset you, or put you at risk.'
- Ask for her cooperation and ideas – 'I need your help to work out the plan. What are your ideas?'

5. **Identify three ways in which you could begin to include patients more in their care.**

Three ways that you could begin to include patients more in their care are:

- Make the best of what you have – if you are routinely working with patients, they are a good source of information and experience. There is often no need to look further if your aim is to improve everyday patient experience.
- Plan well in advance – it may be tempting to leap in and get on with it, but time devoted to planning is well spent.

- Be honest – involvement can go wrong if people believe that they are being invited to explore a wide range of possibilities, or to make decisions, when there are really only a couple of options that can be implemented. Be careful what you ask. If you ask patients if they would like a hot meal in the evening and that is not possible, you will be setting up a situation where the patients can end up feeling disregarded.

- Use the results – just asking for opinions is not enough. Patients and the public will expect changes as a result of their involvement.

- Take it seriously –there needs to be a genuine commitment, not a tick-box philosophy.

Chapter Eight

1. **List four advantages to an organisation of having communities of practice.**

   The advantages of having communities of practice in an organisation are:

   For members:

   - Short-term value: avoids reinventing the wheel; helps with challenges; provides access to expertise; increases confidence; is a non-threatening forum in which to play with ideas

   - Long-term value: personal development; professional development and enhanced identity; network, sharing, generates new knowledge

   For the organisation:

   - Short-term value: early warning system for potential opportunities and threats; time saving, problem solving, knowledge sharing; reuse of resources

   - Long-term-value: innovation; retention of talent; strategic learning; creates a knowledge-sharing culture.

2. **Identify six key qualities for a future 'boss'.**

   Key qualities of a boss are:

   - a sound ethical compass – good people like to work for an organisation that values their trust

- the ability to make difficult decisions – many judgements are made on incomplete information; this will mean mistakes, risk and upset but a decision is better than no decision

- clarity and focus – extracting the crucial point from complexity is essential for achieving an effective strategy so too is the ability to screen out noise and focus on what really matters

- ambition – the best leaders want to create something that outlasts them

- effective communication skills – presenting a vision clearly requires a persuasive leader who can inspire trust and convey authenticity

- the ability to judge people – judging who will work best and where is a key task needing experience and intuition

- a knack for developing talent – people learn a lot from a good mentor, all leaders need to be teachers

- emotional self-confidence – self-confidence enables you to admit your limitations and ask help from colleagues without losing their respect

- adaptability – the ability to reframe and reshape problems increases the chances of a flexible response

- charm – few get to the top without it.

   (adapted from A Survey of Corporate Leadership, *The Economist*, 2003)

3. **What would be the key aspects of culture that would need to be in place to foster a high-performance workplace?**

   The key aspects of culture that would need to be in place to foster a high-performance workplace are:

   - structures – no single organisational structure is seen to be 'best'; consistent features are flatter structures and matrix working

   - processes – minimal processes (i.e. only essential ones); processes that are in place are kept simple; strong communication up and down and across the organisation

   - communication – good communication throughout the organisation, between all groups; managers openly share relevant information with individuals and staff bodies; knowledge is shared

   - leadership – open, visible and accessible.

Index